DIET IS A
4
LETTER WORD

DIET IS A 4 LETTER WORD

SUZIE HEYMAN

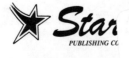

Star
PUBLISHING CO

The following trademarks appear throughout this book: Master Card, Visa, Jello, Hershey's Kisses, Oreo, Saks Fifth Avenue, Macy's, Bloomingdale's, Nutra-Sweet, Opti-Fast, Herbalife, Cambridge, Liquid Protein, Express Mail, IBM, U-Haul, Disney World, Band-Aid, Stuckey, Howard Johnson, Ben & Jerry, Sara Lee, Kentucky Fried Chicken, Neiman-Marcus, Dole-Whip.

For further information: Starlight Publishing Company, Inc.
1893 N.E. 164 Street, Suite 100
North Miami Beach, FL 33162-4109
Telephone (305) 944-8446

Library of Congress Catalog Card Number: 89-051575

ISBN: 0-962468-0-2

This book is dedicated to
ALL the foods I've loved
before...**AND CAN AGAIN!**

and

to my Howard...

Your faith, support and
generosity made this
book...and our terrific
life together...possible.

CONTENTS

PART II — JOURNEY TO FREEDOM

PART III — THE FAT LADY SINGS

PART IV — THE LIFESTYLER

PART V — END OF THE TUNNEL

AFTERWORD

ACKNOWLEDGEMENTS

Without Judy Newell, this book would never have been written. It is Judy's talent and winning spirit that gave me the opportunity to make my dream a reality. I'll always be grateful to you for choosing me as your partner—but most of all, Judy—I want to thank you for being my friend.

A very special thanks goes to Eileen Cypress, M.D., for giving her time and effort to develop THE LIFESTYLER. Through her expertise and guidance, the program is flexible, interesting—and most important—healthy.

To my family goes my appreciation for being such wonderful "book material"...and for EVERYTHING that you are to me. No way, I could get through life without each one of you...and no way, I would want to.

With a great deal of love and respect, I'd like to pay tribute to my mother and dad. It saddens me greatly that they are not here to read this book. However, I'm sure that they would be very proud of me for having the courage to write it.

Buford, you get the credit for helping me discover that THIN truly comes from the inside out—and not from the outside in.

A very special word of recognition for Judy Richman. You always provide the laughter! It's you, Ju, who can yank me up from the depths of despair and point me in the right direction when I get off the track. No one ever had a better *proofreader* or a more delightful friend!

Esther Wolmer, how can I ever thank you for being my "sidekick" from day one? Your faith and support kept me going many times when I was ready to throw in the towel.

From Rock Creek to the last chapter of this book...I've counted on you...and you've been there.

And, I acknowledge—with love, respect, and gratitude—all the members of the THIN WEIGH. You are my friends, my inspiration, my motivation. You—each in your own way —provide me with an abiding faith that one day we will succeed.

PREFACE

I spent the majority of my life dieting. I can't really remember a time when I didn't carry the burden of losing weight on my back. I tried every diet known to mankind. If I didn't try it—it simply means that I had never heard of it.

Sure, I lost weight....tons! But, the minute the diet was over, I returned to my pattern of uncontrollable eating. I hated myself. My fantasy was that I could slip into a coma for six-months and wake up THIN. I even considered robbing a bank to get the money for plastic surgery. I figured I'd keep my hair and change the rest!

Every morning, I promised myself that I'd stay on my diet and I went to sleep hating myself every night for breaking that promise. I suffered pain, shame, and humiliation. I called myself every imaginable name—cheater, weakling, imbecile, pig. My knees got weak at the sight of a scale and my greatest fear was that a salesperson would offer to help me try on clothes and catch a glimpse of my thunder thighs. Of course, I lied about my weight on my driver's license!

I finally stopped dieting. I had to. My health required that I lose weight and keep it off. In my search for a solution to that problem, I made an amazing discovery. Diets NEVER work. They can't. There is a flaw in their concept. My FAT wasn't all my fault. Deprivation has no place to go, but back to overeating. In addition, dieting required perfection—and perfection is not attainable. Dieting led me to failure, self-hatred, and despair. Not dieting led me to freedom.

In an effort to solve my weight problem, I began a fact finding mission to discover more information about food, nutrition, behaviors, and attitudes. I stumbled across a new concept...a new attitude toward food...and toward myself. I stopped dieting and lost sixty-seven pounds.

My purpose for writing this book is to tell you the truth about dieting and the multi-billion dollar industry that feeds on the desperation and despair of overweight people. I'd like to share my new concept with you as you have the right to know that you are entitled to a better way of life. There is no need for you to spend your life trapped in the world of diets. YOU HAVE A CHOICE!

You can conquer your obsession with food—learn to trust your own judgements—differentiate hunger from your emotions. You can develop self-esteem and love yourself more than you love your food. You can become the STAR of your life.

Suzie Heyman

INTRODUCTION

In my medical practice, I am always amazed when I see an overweight patient who is desperately trying to lose weight for a class reunion, a wedding, a family get-together, or any one of the hundreds of other reasons why people want to look thin.

It still astonishes me that an overwhelming majority of dieters are motivated only by cosmetic reasons and very few are concerned with the health problems associated with being overweight. It really should not surprise me. I was once one of those people, who wanted to lose weight to wear a slim knitted suit to a special family party. Although I am a doctor, I wasn't inspired by the fact that those extra fifty-five pounds were reducing my life expectancy.

I knew that being overweight placed me at an increased risk for heart disease, diabetes, high blood pressure, gall bladder disease, gall stones, joint problems, varicose veins, blood clots, and certain forms of cancer.

Like most of you reading this book, I tried to diet a hundred times and managed to lose thousands of pounds in my lifetime. I ate cottage cheese, eggs, spinach, and grapefruit. I drank gallons of water—rigidly weighed and measured every morsel of food I consumed—only to be frustrated by regaining all the lost weight with a few more pounds for good measure.

When I became determined to find a permanent solution to my weight problem, I did extensive reading about food, nutrition, metabolism, and behavior. During the year it took me to lose my fifty-five pounds, slowly, but surely, I gained greater insight into the ideas and concepts involved in helping me formulate a new approach to weight loss. What

I learned is that dieting is truly a ridiculous concept. Depriving oneself over a long period of time can only lead to feelings of deprivation which then trigger bingeing.

I discovered that I didn't need a diet. What I needed was a new lifestyle and not a restricted diet program that I had no hope of following for more than a short time. I realized that food was not the problem. It was what I was doing with the food that kept me fat.

Therefore, I had to learn to differentiate between hunger and anger, stress, boredom, and all the other situations that I perceived as hunger. I had to respond to those situations appropriately and not with food.

It is now twelve years later. I am a thinner, a healthier—and of course,—a happier person. Best of all, I have stopped committing suicide with my knife and fork.

I know this book will give you the insight that you need to understand the problems that have caused you to be overweight. It is important that you believe that you can eat ALL foods—if you learn the techniques to eat them in control. You do not have to look forward to a lifetime of eating pre-packaged food, ridiculous combinations of foods, or avoiding "forbidden" foods forever in an effort to be thin.

Above all, losing weight can add years to your life. And, you will be free to enjoy those years without the restrictions that have always been placed on you. You can finally be in control of what you do with your food and with your life.

EILEEN CYPRESS, M.D.
Miami, Florida

PART I

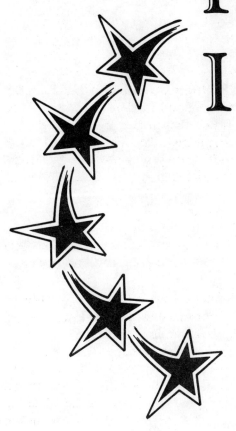

WISH
ON
A STAR

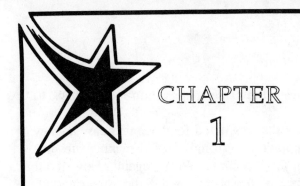

CHAPTER
1

BORN FAT

I was born FAT. My mother took me home from the hospital, gave me a few days off for good behavior, put me on a diet, and there I stayed until I found THE THIN WEIGH!

There has never been a diet I didn't try, always looking for the *magic* to allow me to eat everything I wanted...and still be THIN. Nothing ever worked for me though, because if a diet said, "You have to eat this"—I *hated* it! But, if a diet said, "You can't have this"—I *wanted* it! I was never happy or comfortable with food...or with myself.

When I was ON, I deprived myself of all the foods I enjoyed. When I was OFF, I punished myself for being bad or weak...for cheating and being out of control...and hating myself for my weakness. There was no middle ground—it was black or it was white.

I spent most of my life on this vicious cycle...not finding peace in the eating world...or joy in the DIET WORLD. I figured I was doomed to live my entire life on that roller coaster and destined to lose the battle to be THIN.

Every time I went on a diet and lost weight, I not only gained it back...I gained it back with a <u>BONUS</u>. It didn't matter if I lost the weight rapidly, or if I lost it slowly, the end result was always the same...deprivation led me back to bingeing.

At first, programs that restricted food seemed easy as they eliminated all temptation. Wrong! I tried making substitutions...like *broccoli for chocolate.* Wrong again! How about eating *only* packaged foods to avoid the supermarket, restaurants and other food traps? Still wrong! I tried. I really tried.

To make matters worse, life dealt me a couple of losing hands. For one thing, I had a bout of bad luck with my health. Within the span of a few years, I had several major surgeries (as well as some minor ones), and they made it very difficult for me to keep my life on track. As I felt my life going DOWN the tubes, I saw my weight definitely going UP, UP, UP.

In addition to the problems I was having with my health, other areas of my life were also in chaos. We moved from one area of the city to another, leaving our closest friends behind, and I was lonely. As luck would have it, my kids were at the age when they were becoming independent. *There was no longer any need for Mom to be packing lunches and baking cookies. Sure, what did they care about their poor mother? Now, when I needed them most...they took a powder. Of course, they showed up at mealtime, but could never stay long enough to do the dishes.*

Suddenly, I was on my own to decide what to do with myself. I decided to return to my pre-marriage career. Once, I had been a darn good administrative assistant and thought I could be again. No such luck, I had to leave one job after another because of my health. Nothing in my life was going right!

As I was recovering from *unsuccessful* foot surgery (*surgery #9 in five short years*), the doctors gave me the news that I would need more. Not such terrific news, considering I had been hobbling around for months. The thought of starting over with a new cast, new crutches, and new delays on living my life was the last straw. It made me feel completely hopeless.

What was the use of trying to get myself together when, no matter how hard I tried, I kept running into a brick wall? I hated myself for feeling so useless, and because I hated myself, I took comfort in food...and ATE. I hated my FAT—and myself for being FAT—still, I kept eating and eating and becoming more and more depressed.

I must have appeared even more down in the dumps than usual, when one afternoon my son, Steve, invited my husband and me to go out for a stroll around the mall. I knew it was a sacrifice because Steve <u>hates</u> shopping! We decided to take separate cars and meet there. Then my son could split when he was tired of humoring me instead of sticking around and nagging me to leave when he'd had enough. I was just dragging along, feeling sorry for myself, when all of a sudden, I fell head over heels in love. Sitting in the window of a gift shop was a pig. Yes, a large, pink, overstuffed pig. Granted, he was no Paul Newman or Robert Redford, but there was something about him that made me feel an immediate kinship. He had the biggest grin I had seen in many moons, even though, HE HAD THIGHS JUST LIKE MINE. I wanted that pig!

My husband, Howard, is a truly wonderful man. He is warm, loving and very giving. However, by profession, he's a C.P.A. and, therefore, extremely practical. So, when he saw the price tag on that pig, he suddenly found religion. "What does a Jewish girl need with a $50.00 pig?" Then, dismissing the idea of buying it, he hustled me out of the shop. I was very disappointed. I was upset. I was also

3

leaving the shop with Howard...and without the pig.

I was more depressed than ever, and felt that after all I'd been through lately, you'd think, at least, I'd be entitled to a pig, if I wanted it. But, no matter, the thrill was gone anyway, so we said goodbye to our son and headed home.

We had barely gotten from the car to the house when Steve arrived and HE HAD THE PIG! To my delight, without prompting, nudging or nagging, that wonderful child of mine had bought me that expensive pig...with his own money. *(It didn't matter one bit, I had given him the money just that morning.)*

On the spot, I decided Buford (the name my pig came with) was just what I needed to keep me company during my next surgical ordeal.

The day of my surgery was truly grim. Even though it was only an out-patient procedure, I still had to rise at dawn and drag myself to the hospital. And that wasn't all! I wasn't permitted to eat or drink anything after midnight...not even coffee. And, to make matters worse, it was also the day the University of Miami Hurricanes were to play Boston College and I hated missing that football game! However, since it was getting to be pretty routine for life not to go my way, I went off to the hospital with *"no comment."*

My surgery turned out to be far more successful than the Hurricanes. Later in the day on our way home, Howie and I were able to catch the final moments of the game on the radio. Wait! Maybe things are getting better. Hope grew. Miami was winning! *Forget the cast on my foot, sticking out the back window of the car...a victory could make my day!* Then, just as we pulled into our driveway...it happened! I listened in total disbelief as Doug Flutie threw his incredible *"Hail Flutie"* pass, and Boston College defeated my beloved Hurricanes. I hobbled into the house, deflated, defeated, and depressed...all in all, not a happy camper!

Only Buford cared. He sat on my dresser through all the days and nights I recuperated in bed. Bless him, he really did cheer me up...both amusing and intriguing me. A hundred times a day, I contemplated, "Why is he smiling when he is so FAT? Doesn't he hate himself the way I do?" With plenty of time to ponder, I finally decided that he didn't hate himself because it is appropriate for a pig to be FAT. Then, I wondered, "Could I put a big grin on my face by learning to love my FAT thighs and my FAT self? If it is appropriate for Buford, maybe, just maybe, it is appropriate for me to be FAT." Could it just be my lot in life? Yes, that has to be it! Destiny has spoken. My new mission in life...learn to love myself FAT.

But, my plan never had a chance to be executed because the fates intervened. My Howie failed his "stress test." *What a dummy, I told him to study!* Now, he needed a heart catheterization because the doctors suspected he might have a clogged artery. I was frantic, practically immobilized with fear, at the prospect Howie was facing a heart attack, open heart surgery, or worst of all, possible death. Naturally, I couldn't imagine life without him. *We had such a terrific partnership: He made the money...I spent it, I picked out his clothes...he wore them, I made the trash, he took it out. Sure he snores, but still, I didn't want to lose him.*

The history of his family was not in his favor. His father died from heart disease at the early age of fifty-six. Was my Howie to suffer the same fate? I prayed, "Dear God...NO!"

I was no stranger to watching a loved one recover from heart surgery, so I didn't want that for Howie either. My mother had a valve replacement years before it was in vogue. My cousin, Martin, was only thirty-six when he endured open heart surgery after suffering his heart attack. I couldn't bear the thought of my Howie having to face a similar ordeal.

We were very fortunate as, thank heavens, Howie's "*cath*" showed only a minor obstruction. I listened intently, as his cardiologist sat on the edge of his bed, explaining the requirements for his future care. I wanted to hear every word so I could take **perfect** care of my husband from now on. The doctor advised him, "Get to your ideal weight, restrict foods high in fat, avoid sodium, and exercise thirty minutes every day."

Suddenly, I got a knot in the pit of my stomach as I couldn't ignore the fact the doctor also meant me. I, too, had a very bad family history. My father had his first heart attack at age fifty, and died when he was sixty-two. My mother lost her life to heart disease when she was only sixty-seven years old. There was no question about it, I had been robbed! Not only was I deprived of more time to enjoy my parents, I was heir to their legacy of health problems. At least, that's the way I had always figured it, but after the doctor spoke to Howie...everything changed.

It suddenly became "crystal clear" that the history of my parents did not have to be my fate as well. I could change my future. And, brother, some *MAJOR* changes were necessary. Not only was I about seventy-five pounds over-weight, I ate only junk food, and my favorite form of exercise was walking to the refrigerator. Something drastic had to be done. But what?

I left the hospital in turmoil. Half of me was elated, joyous that my Howie had been spared. *Thank you, God, thank you. Thank you, for not making him suffer and allowing no harm to come to him.* The other half of me was hysterical at the realization that a serious flaw had developed in my plan to live the rest of my life FAT...but happy. I might live happily, but for how long?

That question gave me a very sleepless night. I tossed and turned, trying to sort out everything in my mind. I felt I owed it to Howie and my children to try to take better care of myself and spare them the agony I'd just endured. To heck with that! I owed it to myself! *I knew open heart surgery would certainly yield a room full of flowers, and probably all the candy I could eat, however,* I DID NOT WANT OPEN HEART SURGERY...*or anything like it!*

What could I do to avoid it, though? What was available? Return to the diet club, *even though, I had joined and quit, at least, one thousand times?* Go on a liquid fast, *even though, the taste was so horrible that death seemed like the kinder option?* Go back to pills or shots, *or would that be worse for my health than staying FAT?* What about those packaged or canned foods? No way!

Once, I gave that stuff to my dog, Tagel. He sniffed it, then tried to dig a hole in our ceramic tile floor to bury it. That didn't work, so he walked away, and wouldn't come back 'til that stuff was safely in the garbage. I trust this dog...if he wouldn't eat it, well.....

What could I do? What would work? What? As the dawn broke, I came up with one of my brightest ideas...EVER. Since I was the one who needed to lose the weight, maybe, just maybe, I should do it **MY WAY!**

I was a certified, card carrying expert on DIETING. Certainly, I knew a lot about calories; I had been counting them all my life. For sure, I knew everything about "fattening" foods. They were the ones I loved the most.

WOW!! Lucky me, the opportunity of a lifetime was presenting itself. I would analyze my objectives, outline a plan of action, and stack all the odds in my favor—a "failure proof" system for losing weight. This time, I couldn't afford to fail. (*And, while I was at it, I would rid myself of the guilt,*

depression and despair of being FAT.)
Let's see, what precisely do I want to accomplish?

1) I want to be healthy.
2) I want to eat like a normal person.
3) I want the rest of my life to include
   the foods I love...*especially chocolate.*
4) I want to end the pain of being FAT.

One by one, I analyzed my objectives:

1) To be healthy, I knew I had to sacrifice some of the foods I was eating; *probably my first one hundred favorites. Okay, I'm willing to do that because I want to live.* I suppose that some form of exercise is also going to be necessary. Let's see, I always enjoyed walking *inside* a mall, maybe, it could be as much fun to try it *outside* a mall. Just a second, fun or no fun doesn't matter. Whether I like it or not, I have to do it. *It's just as I used to tell my children, "Nobody asked you to like it, I just asked you to do it."*
2) Wanting to eat like a normal person is going to be a bit tougher. After all, how would I know what a "normal" person ate? I can find out, though. The newsstands are jammed with magazines containing information about food, proper nutrition and health. *I am confident that part is going to be easy.*
3) I didn't want to live the rest of my life without the foods I loved. Sure even a lifelong "junk food junkie" can be rehabilitated, but it has to be within reason. No way will I give up chocolate!! And, why should I? *I didn't design the universe and determine that chocolate would be so terrific and broccoli so*

8

bland. Besides, during all my diet years, I tried substituting broccoli for chocolate, and it NEVER worked anyway. Nothing that led to failure was going to be included in my new plan, and, quite frankly, life without chocolate would surely lead me to failure!
4) Gaining control over food would make the pain go away. Never again, did I want to eat until I was sick to my stomach and...sick of myself.

My aim was to devise a program I could live with—without too many rules—to provide me with a learning experience in the art of control. No longer could I afford to sit around waiting for the **perfect** diet—or the magic pill—to allow me to get THIN. The time for waiting is over. The time for doing is here!

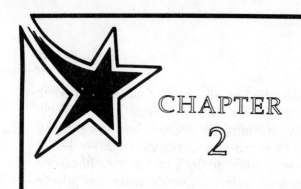

CHAPTER
2

I AIN'T SO BAD

Instinctively, I knew I needed a whole new attitude. I couldn't keep telling myself, "You are a big, FAT, weak-livered cheater with absolutely no willpower and that's why your life is in shambles." Besides, I wasn't sure that was exactly accurate...

I thought about my life, I'm not a flop in everything. In fact, I'm pretty darn good at a whole bunch of things. I am bright and funny. I am good-hearted and caring. I am responsible and faithful. I am honest and fair. Honest and fair? Wait a minute, how honest am I being to discount all my good qualities, and lump myself into one big failure, just because I'm FAT? *After all, can you truly judge a person's self-worth by whether or not she needs liposuction?*

And how fair was I being by just looking at one side of the story? Maybe, it's time for a fresh inventory of the facts.

I was a terrific daughter. No hardship, the job was an easy one to do. My wonderful parents blessed me with their beautiful old-fashioned values and our times together left me with some of the most precious memories of my life.

My father was a wise, practical man, but his attitude toward food was, "It is valuable and should not be wasted." Early on, he enrolled me in the *Clean Plate Club* and expected my membership to be constant and current. Often, Dad spoke of the "starving children in Europe" and urged me to do the patriotic thing by eating my food. *I was just a kid. How could I be expected to make the connection between my overeating and their hunger? No need, I had so much faith in my father, I cleaned my plate on his advice. Now, I'll bet that, at least, part of my thigh problem is due to the sacrifice I made for some hungry child in Poland.*

My mother had a marvelous sense of humor and a special talent for having fun. We were both a tad bit crazy, so much alike, that Howie referred to us as "two flakes in the great snowstorm of life." Her theory, "If you go to a party and it's a dud, you can still have a wonderful time. But, if you go to a wonderful party and you're a dud...forget the wonderful time."

She raised me to be fun-loving and gets the credit for being my inspiration when I decided to make a surprise first birthday party for my dog, Tagel. My concern was that not everyone would understand the need to celebrate this particular occasion. However, since she always encouraged me to seek fun, I made the party.

To this day, my friends and I talk about that party and we all agree it deserves to go into the record books as a winner! I've often worried though that Tagel sniffed around and got wise to the surprise, but he's such a master of deception, I'm sure no one, but me, noticed.

My mom's favorite way to show how much she loved her family was to spend hours cooking all of our favorite dishes. She left little doubt that food was the STAR of our celebrations, and when life didn't go right, she comforted me with *"something delicious."*

11

My Mom and Dad taught me many great values, but if they were here right now, I'd tell them, "Daddy, you were wrong about food. It's better to waste it than suffer the misery of overeating. So, I am tendering my resignation to the *Clean Plate Club.* Mama, I wish I could thank you for all the friendship and love you gave me. It was even better than your fabulous cooking and baking...but your chicken soup sure was close." *Wonderful parents...wonderful daughter!*

Talk about luck...I found my "*Mr. Wonderful.*" You just don't get any luckier than my Howard. He is a fine man, who brings a bit of *sanity* to my life, just as I have added much *craziness* to his. Thankfully through all my "hair brained" schemes, the man treats me as if I am *perfectly normal.*

Once, I put a non-refundable deposit on a new house, which prompted him to mention, "Honey, we already own the house we're living in." My reply, "There is absolutely no need to worry, sweetheart. I'm sure we can sell this house in time." He bought that story! He believed in me! That made me feel so secure, not quite as secure as when we sold our old house...but secure!

It's possible I'm not a **perfect** wife and, Lord knows, we certainly have had our share of rough times. Luckily, none of that matters, as during our twenty-nine terrific years together, he continues to love me...even with my one or two minor flaws. *Good score as a wife.*

And, of course, SUPER MOM. Sure, my three kids are all college grads now, but I raised them from *scratch*...they were just babies when I gave birth to them. Gosh, I love those kids! Just the mere thought of them fills me with such pride I could easily burst. They got my maximum effort always: never missed a car pool; baked better cookies than any other mother in the neighborhood; helped with homework (*except math*); and always volunteered to have their New Year's Eve parties in our house.

Looking back, I wonder how I even managed to survive. Barbara was a three year old and Janet a mere thirteen months when the stork delivered Steve. Diapers, formulas and toilet training! I don't know how I made it through those days, and I didn't even have the brains to ask for help. It was <u>my</u> job, so I did it, because even when it's tough, you still have to do it...if it's <u>your</u> job.

Early on, we made a commitment to our kids to provide love, values, a college education, a new car, and a free Sunday dinner for life. *I'm not cooking much these days, but <u>every</u> Sunday a gourmet meal appears on the table. I may <u>never</u> be elected "Mother of the Year," but I am in the running for "Queen of Take-Out."*

In return, our children have blessed us with abundant joy, the happiest times of our lives, and an immeasurable sense of accomplishment; living proof that the most important benefits in life come from hard work and commitment. *High score for motherhood.*

Family to me includes...siblings, nieces, and nephews. While my folks were alive, every Sunday we spent the day with them, together with my sister, Eileen, and her husband, Bobby, and their kids, Marlene and Stanley. After my folks passed away, we continued the family tradition.

Our children grew up together, getting the best of both worlds. My sister provides my kids with the sensible approach, "Study hard and save your money." On the other hand, her kids could count on me for the opportunity to share in any wild excursion. *"Mar, let's blow your allowance and go shopping. Stan, remember if you need a couple of extra bucks for the movies, I'm in!"*

13

Unfortunately, my younger sister, Kate, moved away when she married Larry. No problem, I found a way to spoil her kids, Jason and Rachel, via long distance telephone and Express Mail. *Pretty good score there...good sister...great aunt!*

If you're looking for terrific friends...I've got them. In my happy times and in my sorrow, they are with me. I hope, in return, I've left no doubt that they can always count on me. Life would be a "bummer" without them...and absolutely no fun! Oh sure, I often acknowledge how lucky I am to have them. You know what? They aren't so bad off either to have me for a friend. *Another good score...for friendship.*

Unique is the word for my employment history. Finding a job...no problem! Liking it...another matter. At one point, I changed jobs so often Howard assured me, "When we file our tax return, we'll need a cardboard box to send your W-2's to the government." *"So what, Howard? Are you suggesting I settle for less than living up to my maximum potential?"*

Boy, my personal inventory was going fabulously well. The more I audited, the more I learned...and the more I liked myself!

Who says I'm a flop as a daughter, a wife, a mother, a sister, an aunt, a friend, or an employee? Nothing in my life seems to be out of control, except my relationship with food, and therein lies the discovery that led me to THE THIN WEIGH.

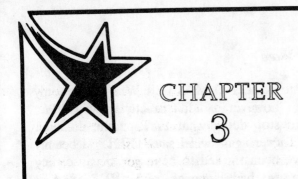

CHAPTER 3

GROW UP AND BE THIN

What a revelation! I'm not a flop as a person! Still, there is nothing respectable about my failure as a dieter. No matter, I don't have that worry anymore. From this day forward, diets are a thing of the past. The time has come for me to be independent, get to my ideal weight...and STAY THERE. Carefully, I considered what to do next. No way I can fail...this time, my life is at stake...

I reviewed the problems of the past for clues:

> 1. Losing weight had never been FAST enough.
> 2. Losing weight had been very TOUGH.

Time to grow up! FAST or SLOW, TOUGH OR EASY, it still has to be done...nobody promised me a *"rose garden."* If I want to be THIN, independent, free, and reach my ideal weight, I need an open-ended, realistic goal. My statement for success:

> *"I AM GOING TO MY IDEAL WEIGHT...NO MATTER HOW LONG IT TAKES...NO MATTER HOW TOUGH IT IS!"*

15

Oh, I am going to do it...NO MATTER WHAT...the only problem remaining, however, I didn't exactly know HOW. For sure, I had to stop doing what FAT people do...diet. This is a new era...never again will I say, "DIET." I bet my parents would have been thrilled to hear that because they didn't like me to use bad language, and...**DIET IS A 4 LETTER WORD!**

I am going to be free...free to control myself...free to make my own choices and still lose weight. I'll simply remember the bottom line...I WANT TO BE THIN.

I became a detective, tracking down clues to help identify my eating behaviors and didn't even know then that I was hot on the trail of the <u>real</u> criminal. I always just assumed food is the villain—not true—it's attitude that's the culprit! That's right, it's in the <u>head</u> and not in the stomach.

I first discovered I hated mornings and everything about them, especially breakfast. The thought of eating food in the A.M. gagged me. Eat it? I didn't even want to think about it. Yet, breakfast was a requirement of the DIET WORLD. Not this time! *Well, maybe, just a tiny breakfast...no reason to get too defiant! So, as sort of a compromise, I decided that perhaps it was best to have one slice of thin toast with coffee. No sense taking unnecessary chances from day one.*

Lunch time wasn't a particularly hungry time for me either. The problem was the food conversations I conducted in my head all morning. "What am I going to eat and when am I going to eat it?" And, then there was menu fantasy, "Shall I have the Chinese, Italian, Deli, Tacos? What?" *My intellect told me that twenty-five hours a day was just too long for food to be talking to me. Besides food really cannot talk, and it was time to admit, I had simply been talking to myself.*

No matter, I needed a solution. So, henceforth, 1:00 P.M. would be my lunch time. What's more, it would also be a good idea to prepare my lunches in advance. I rushed to the grocery store, making an unusual "*cameo*" appearance. (*I hate to go food shopping and try to avoid it at all costs!*) I bought loaves and loaves of thin sliced bread and tons of turkey salami. Then, I made stacks of sandwiches and loaded them into my freezer.

Ignoring the past advice of the DIET WORLD, "Eat variety...*tuna fish, cottage cheese, salad, turkey*," I got brave and made all the sandwiches turkey salami. So what, if they are all the same? It's **MY CHOICE!** I can skip variety if I want to. *Besides, when I'm not dieting, I usually eat regular salami on regular bread every day. Know why? I like it!.*

Okay, now lunch is handled...onward to dinner! We had always eaten dinner very early because during tax season, Howard had to return to his office. That situation offered me the opportunity to have a second dinner when Howie came home. Oh, I may as well be honest. The truth is from the time he left the house, it was one long meal all night long. Deciding to eat dinner later would win only half the battle and, accordingly, I made a vow, "I will have only <u>ONE</u> snack after dinner."

In addition, some heavy duty portion control was also in order. I had a FAT brain as well as a FAT stomach. My old program was to eat "family style"—*for a family of five, that is.* Perish the thought I'd ever stop short of finishing all that was available for eating, even if there was so much food it made me feel sick...physically and emotionally!

Thus, another hurried trip to the grocery store (*oh, how I hated that!*) to buy a variety of every frozen diet dinner known to man. Gaining control over food was my top priority, and if the entire DIET WORLD claimed that the contents of that little box was an appropriate portion, it must be so. After all, aren't they the experts on portion control?

17

I'll never know how I managed to survive the shock of seeing what they consider a portion for a grown up. To tell the truth, I used to eat more than that putting the leftovers away after a dinner party! *After seeing their "spaghetti dinner" and NOT going into cardiac arrest, I felt better about being in danger of an impending heart attack and had much greater faith in the strengths of my cardio-vascular system.*

I wanted to lose weight all right, but I didn't want to die of malnutrition, so to my magnificent frozen feast, I added a baked potato...*a very small one*. Even though I didn't have to follow the rules of the past anymore, the potato still made me feel <u>very</u> guilty.

To my great surprise, soon I was handling the portion, handling the guilt, and losing weight. Imagine that! Eating my own way and losing weight, too. Maybe I was on to something!

The only problem left unsolved was my *beloved chocolate.* After a lifetime of dieting, I was much too brainwashed to walk over to a piece of candy...and eat it. Talk about being blessed...I thanked my lucky stars to be living in the *Age of Nutra Sweet.* Surely, I could fill the bill for chocolate and not have to stoop to eating bad foods. I'll simply select a diet product—something I can trust—diet chocolate pudding. *After all, if you can't trust Jello and Bill Cosby, who can you trust?* There, it's settled! One portion of pudding every night after dinner. JUST ONE?

Instinctively, I knew the secret of success was learning to eat ONE portion. It had to be! Eating **ALL** or **NONE** never worked. This was scary!! What if I couldn't settle for ONE? Then what would happen? I analyzed my options and made a few simple rules:

Rule 1. If I can control it, I can have it.
Rule 2. If I can't control it, I can't have it.
Rule 3. If I can't control it and I have it,
       I CAN'T BE THIN.

So I began eating one portion of pudding every night, choosing 9:00 P.M. as snack time, to eliminate the mental argument, "Should I have it now or should I have it later?" *A specific time for eating was critical to stop me from thinking about food from the minute I finished dinner until the minute I fell asleep at night.* My plan was to finish dinner around 7:00 P.M. and just wait until 9:00 P.M. to have my pudding. Sounds pretty easy! WRONG! It's far from easy, but it's possible, and I was going to do it...NO MATTER WHAT!

Many a night the waiting seemed almost unbearable, especially when Howard was working, as food had always been such wonderful company for me. I tried to keep busy, so there was some good news. I finally finished the afghan I started for my sister's twenty-first birthday...*not bad considering she's only forty-two!* I read a little, watched TV, took a shower, played with my dog, anything to occupy my time. But when 9:00 P.M. arrived, I won the "gold medal" for racing to the fridge for my pudding. I ate it SLOWLY, knowing there was another twenty-four hours before I'd have more.   My brain was taking my stomach to school and teaching it "CONTROL 101."

I pondered some of the other behaviors that led me astray. They, too, needed solutions or the old programs of the past would lead me to repeating the bad habits of a lifetime—for a lifetime—and that wasn't what I wanted.

Meals were not really a big problem for me. After dinner was when I had the trouble. For example, I could polish off five pounds of turkey simply because it was left on the

19

frame. I felt it was my duty to pick at any food that was available for eating... until it was gone. Why? Why was it my duty? THIN people didn't feel that need, but how did they avoid it? I watched them and discovered: THIN people put all the food they plan to eat on their own plate. They eat as much as they want—then put down their knife and fork—and never eat another bite. Hurrah! I found my new THIN behavior.

Because my food must be on my plate I developed a very amusing morning routine! My kitchen is not too large, *(big enough, of course, considering how much I use it)* therefore, my freezer and my toaster are very close to each other. I open the door of the freezer and take out a piece of bread. I put it in the toaster, open the door of the pantry, and take out a plate. The toast pops up, I put it on my plate, put a tad of diet margarine on it, pick it up...and eat it. Then, I open the door of the dishwasher and put the plate in it. Know why I need the plate? It reminds my brain, that it's my food...because it's on my plate!

Putting my food on a plate also helps avoid the nightmare of eating anything out of its original container. Once, I took a quart of ice cream and a spoon with me to watch T.V. I only planned to eat a scoop, honest. *At the first taste of the delicious ice cream, I suffered "total amnesia" and forgot to stop eating—until I wound up with an empty carton!*

Every time I discovered another of my "behavior problems," I looked for a workable solution. Soon, I really was taking control of my portions, and delightfully disproving many of the *"diet facts"* I'd lived with for so many years. With all my heart, I had truly believed that a "good dieter," NEVER ate "forbidden" foods (no cheating allowed) and ALWAYS lost weight FAST...and the ONLY true measure of success was the scale! What baloney! Once I put all that "stuff" on the back burner I finally found what had eluded me for so long...control!

CHAPTER
4

BEAM ME UP

A FAST weight loss was no longer my main concern. A THIN LIFESTYLE was far more satisfactory to me than going "on and off" a new diet every week. I was comfortable with my choices and my aim was to get to my ideal weight...and stay there forever! No doubt in my mind...THERE IS NO BRASS RING ON THE DIET MERRY-GO-ROUND. The brass ring is finding the middle ground...

Replacing the negatives of the DIET WORLD, with a positive attitude, allowed me to take each day as a learning experience—practicing my new way of eating—making the best choices possible—and enjoying my new found freedom. Whenever I had a temporary lapse, I didn't berate myself, or call myself the names of the past..."bad, cheater, stupid, imbecile, or pig."

I just reinforced my belief, "You are still learning and it is going to take time, patience, and practice to become a THIN person." Since I knew I was NEVER going back to my old way of eating—and this was it for life—what was my hurry? Best of all, success meant NEVER having to suffer through the despair of failing on another diet and that was worth fighting for.

Success gave me confidence. It gave me hope. It gave me faith. It gave me curiosity!

All of a sudden, I wanted to know more about THIN people. Up until now, I never knew anything about them. How could I? Frankly, in the past, I never liked them very much. Besides, I was jealous! After all, they were THIN, and I had been cursed...with FAT.

I did a "quick study" on THIN folks. To my amazement, I discovered THIN has absolutely nothing to do with "*luck* or *curses*." THIN people have no magic formula for success. All they have is a different *relationship* with food. There is no secret to their automatic control. In fact, it even has a name...*meals. That sure does explain why I knew nothing about it. What FAT person has time for meals? Not I! I woke up in the morning and started eating and continued eating until I went to sleep at night.*

There's more: THIN people eat as much food as they need, then they stop eating, feeling no obligation to eat everything in sight, or anything they don't enjoy. Amazing! Furthermore for some reason, they are also comfortable with food and trust their ability to make choices.

THIN people don't binge eat. Know why? They don't have room for so much food. THIN people don't eat food they hate in an effort to manipulate a number on a scale. THIN people don't eat food to prevent it from spoiling. THIN people are not ashamed to eat in public. THIN people eat consciously...aware of what they eat and why they eat it. THIN people never **reward** or **punish** themselves with dessert.

THIN is what I truly wanted to be—in mind—as well as in body...free of guilt and out of pain. I wanted to call my own shots and not feel like a criminal every time I ate something that wasn't on the "approved list" of the DIET WORLD.

Let's be honest, I wanted *real* chocolate! Why couldn't I have it? Why was it considered a bad food, anyway? In truth, can food really be **good** or **bad**? Did certain foods truly have power over me? Were there actually foods that made me FAT...and foods that didn't? Did I have to eat frozen diet dinners for the rest of my life to be THIN? *Scotty, maybe it's time to beam me up! All of a sudden, everything I have always believed seems extremely illogical.*

Food didn't have more power than I did. How could it? It had no way to get into my mouth without my help. If I chose not to eat it, it had no choice but to just sit on my plate. And, what if I wanted to banish it to the garbage disposal, there was no way it could *beg for mercy*!

To heck with you, DIET WORLD, the time has come for me to make ONLY my own choices. I feel ready to take full responsibility for myself...to eat EVERYTHING in measurable portions. *My intelligence warned me that all foods are not created equal. Obviously, the more calories something has, the less of it you can eat. That makes sense: The bigger the portion, the smaller the weight loss, but can it be that simple? It sounds too good to be true!*

Maybe, there was no truth to the fact that some foods are *fattening* and some are not. Maybe the secret is simply to learn how much of each food to eat. Maybe, just maybe, the DIET WORLD is wrong and there is no *magic* formula for losing weight. Is it possible the DIET WORLD is a fraud? *Is it possible I could get burned at the stake for asking these questions?*

WOW! How fortunate! Again, I've stumbled across something BIG! However, it's a mixed bag...terrific news, if I can handle the responsibility, but a bit frightening. Never again will I be able to blame the Gods or curse the fates for making me FAT. Never again will I be able to wish on the first star to be THIN. *Cursing or wishing just won't make me THIN!* If I want to be THIN, I will have to get THIN.

Giving up wishing was going to be tough. My earliest birthday memory is when I turned five...the same year we moved from Brooklyn to Miami Beach. My mother made me a party in the lobby of our apartment house and baked me a beautiful birthday cake. With the candles glowing, I made my wish, *"Let me be THIN like the other girls."* Then, I blew out the candles and cut myself a <u>big</u> piece of cake. I was doing two things wrong:

1. Wishing to be THIN
2. Eating a <u>big</u> piece of cake.

From now on, it will be a <u>small</u> piece of cake as that will help make my wish come true.

My new plan is to love **myself** more than I love my next meal. Food, you have been the STAR of my life long enough. Move over, I am going to replace you. Sorry, but you've lost the role to someone more qualified to play it! From this day forward, it's THE SUZIE HEYMAN STORY, starring Suzie Heyman. I am no longer a lost cause, or a rebel without a cause, I have a new cause...ME!

I wanted a symbol of my new found freedom and, thank heavens, jewelry has no calories. I rushed out and bought myself a pin...a rhinestone STAR. *Granted, it was a bit tacky, but I ignored that fact, pinned it to my shoulder, and have worn a STAR every day since.* It reminds me that <u>indeed</u> I AM THE STAR OF MY OWN LIFE.

Now, I have a marvelous STAR collection that numbers about one hundred different STARS. Of course I like them all, but, forever, I think my favorite will be the gold and diamond pendant I bought when I lost my fiftieth pound. That STAR helped me make a big statement, "I'm entitled to be proud of myself and I'm entitled to say so." *Can you think of a better way to make a positive statement than with gold and diamonds?* It's a tough fight to be the STAR of your own life, but it's worth it!

CHAPTER
5

NOT GUILTY, YOUR HONOR

Getting success in my sights thrilled me. I decided to fight for control for the rest of my life; yet, there remained one obstacle: GUILT! As a result of being "born and bred" in the DIET WORLD, I accepted as common knowledge that there was a Forbidden City...a place where I would never be permitted to dwell. The thought of letting go of that idea made me feel very uncomfortable. The mere mention of eating and enjoying bad foods seemed decadent...

However, if FOOD IS JUST FOOD, then why do I have to avoid the most delicious? THIN people eat them! Why then, if they are just like other foods, did they always lead to the destruction of my diet? Why did they always blow my control?

Let's examine other items that are "forbidden." There definitely is a certain mystique that surrounds them, but is it simply because they are "forbidden?"

I wonder, "Do you think if Joanne Woodward gave me permission to pursue my secret passion for Paul Newman, it would become less exciting?" (Believe me when I tell you, "I'd give my eye teeth...and a whole lot more...to find out.") Okay, Howie, now you know the truth about the only secret I've ever kept from you. Not only am I madly in love with Paul, but

I've kept his picture under my pillow for the last thirty years. Are you leaving me or are you going to be a good sport about this?

Perhaps, my best bet is to concentrate on "forbidden" foods. If food is no longer "forbidden" can fear be eliminated? Can choice replace guilt? Can my THIN LIFE-STYLE teach me to eat ANY food in control? *Can I get FAT from just thinking this way?* It is certainly worth an investigation...

Although, I was quite satisfied with the diet pudding, my heart still yearned for real chocolate...the chocolate of my youth: HERSHEY'S. Could it be, was it safe to even consider that I could eat it? Just the thought filled me with overwhelming guilt.

Truly, I felt like Public Enemy Number One as I pursued my investigation by reading the back of a box of diet pudding. To my amazement, I discovered that one half cup...my portion...had ninety calories. It was much more than I expected, but, still, could it help me? I was sure even one HERSHEY'S KISS (*so precious and delicious*) must have hundreds and hundreds of calories. If not, why was it "forbidden?" Want to hear something astonishing? I found that one kiss has only twenty-five calories and, all this time, I had been eating sixty-five more calories to use a diet product. *Shame on you Bill Cosby, you should have told me!*

What a bombshell! I could actually eat the candy and save sixty-five calories. A MAJOR MIRACLE!

I rushed to the grocery store (*this time, I almost enjoyed going*), bought a carload of kisses and hurried home to eat the first one. (*No eating in the car...not a good behavior.*) I unwrapped it with shaking hands...and ate it SLOWLY. It was heaven...until I got the guilt attack. Candy—I was eating candy—*real* candy! Immediately, I thought, "You better give up the idea of losing weight. The only thing you are losing right now is your mind." **BAD, BAD, BAD.** Hey, wait a minute. Remember...

Rule 1: If you can control it, you can have it.

I'm only eating ONE. That's control. That's tough. That's another miracle! I knew that the guilt would destroy me if I didn't get rid of it. If I feel guilty about eating ONE piece of candy, it will surely lead me to finishing the package.

It was like robbing a bank! Who, in their right mind, would go into a bank, pull a gun on a teller, and demand a dollar? If it's bad to rob a bank, you might as well take ALL the money while you're at it. If eating candy is bad, guilt would lead me to a binge. You simply can't get any *"badder"* than bad.

Getting rid of that guilt was urgent or I would forfeit the opportunity to make my own choices. Where in the world did I get all this guilt anyway? Simple! It was a gift from the DIET WORLD. Suddenly, it hit me: Diets were designed to control me...instead of allowing me the opportunity to control myself.

There's nothing wrong with eating candy in CONTROL! DIET WORLD, that's just your opinion! And, who are you anyway to set yourself up as judge and jury of what foods can be *controlled* and what foods are *uncontrollable*? Now, I'm angry! Damn it, while I had been fighting so hard to stop food from controlling me, I had foolishly allowed the DIET WORLD to control me instead. Well, forget it, no more! DIET WORLD...thanks, but no thanks...I CAN CONTROL MYSELF.

I will never again reach for a bag of *cucumbers* or *carrots* to replace a piece of *candy*. There's no question about it—a small portion of something you like is much better then a whole lot of something you don't enjoy. Goodbye, DIET WORLD...I am packing up and leaving. Goodbye, guilt...I don't need you any more either. I ran to Macy's and bought the largest gift box that was available. Hurriedly, I packed up <u>ALL</u> my guilt, wrapped it, and sent it Express Mail to Opti-Fast.

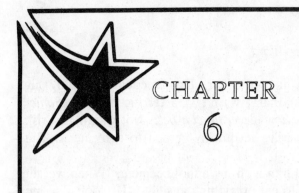

CHAPTER
6

HAPPY DAYS

My positive attitude was working, and it led me to believe I had actually won the war over food. After all, every day I ate one chocolate kiss...and it tasted like victory to me. Three cheers! I WAS CURED! No way! I was overlooking the strongest tie of all; the one that had kept me bound to food for the majority of my life: **FEELINGS.** Sure, everything was fine when everything was fine, but...

One rainy Sunday morning, I awoke in a blue funk. Nothing felt right with the world. I wasn't even sure why— nor did I care— because I knew <u>exactly</u> how to fix it. Just head to my favorite mall, go directly to the food court, and eat one of everything available! After all, if there is anything better for a blue funk than shopping, it's gotta be eating!

I mused, "Maybe, I should start with dessert 'cause life is so uncertain. You never know and what if...heaven forbid...a sudden hurricane comes through town?"

The thought of the binge made me anxious to get going, so I rushed my husband along. Of course, at that point, I didn't bother to mention to him that the mall I wanted to go to was way across town. I felt blue, I had a binge coming, and that was all that mattered. Besides, my Howie wouldn't mind; he'd take me, I bet he would...or else!

When we got into the car, Howie could judge by my charming manner that I wasn't in a terrific mood. (*Sometimes I marvel at how clever he can be*). Not wanting to risk his life unnecessarily, he quickly agreed to take me to The Galleria.

Then I zapped him with my announcement, "When we get there, I'm going to eat everything in sight." He looked at me amazed and asked, "Where did this behavior suddenly come from?" Honestly, he tried very hard to dissuade me, "Honey you've worked so hard to come this far and I'm so proud of the courage you've shown up to now"...but to no avail. Nothing he said budged me, "I don't care about any of that. I'm adamant! Don't you understand, I don't feel well? I have a binge coming to me and, no matter what you say, I'm going to have it."

After that on the long drive to the mall, Howard played it safe by not talking to me. Instead, he pushed my favorite cassette into the tape player...*One Voice* by Barbra Streisand. (*Maybe, if I could sing like her, I wouldn't mind being FAT?*)

While visions of sugar plums danced in my head, Barbra started singing, *Happy Days Are Here Again.* My mind drifted back to the happy days of my life—or the days that should have been happy...

In high school, I was voted *Most Likely to Succeed;* won the Leadership Award; served as Editor-in-Chief of the yearbook and a member of the Student Council. Not bad, nothing to be ashamed of. In fact, I was feeling mighty proud of myself until I remembered how the pretty, fluffy, THIN girls never invited me to join their cliques or clubs. I assumed they didn't think I was good enough just because I was FAT...and I agreed! Nothing else matters if you are FAT...but, somehow, FAT always matters. *Not such happy school days, Ms. Streisand.*

32

So what? Thank the good Lord, one of my diets actually worked the year my "Prince Charming" came along. At our wedding, I couldn't have been happier—THIN and married—what an unbeatable combination! It doesn't get any better. *Looking back, it probably was a mistake to head for the buffet after the ceremony. With my first bite of food, I started gaining all my weight back.*

Married life suited me fine and, immediately, we began our family. Believe it or not, we produced three children in a span of three years. I was pregnant so often, I didn't have time to worry about being FAT. Quickly, our blessings included two beautiful daughters and the magical moment when our son was born. Two girls and a boy, for sure, now, I had it all. Gosh, it can't get any better than that.

The happiness I felt at the birth of my son was short lived. I felt ecstatic only until it was time to go home from the hospital. Stupidly, I had packed a pre-pregnancy dress to wear home and it didn't even come close to buttoning. *Gee Barbra, again not such a happy day.*

Now, my depression was worse than ever. Certainly, I must have had some happy days I can think about. If not, I should have chosen a mall closer to home and spared myself this long horrible drive. *Damn you FAT, you always find a way to spoil everything! Remember all the invitations that I never accepted because of you, and worse yet, the horror of accepting and going to a party ashamed of myself? True, every now and again, I got lucky, when one of my diet successes coincided with a special occasion, but not often enough.*

Barbra, why are you singing this painful song today anyway? I don't like to think about my FAT days. Instead, I'll concentrate on one of the happiest days ever...the day my Barbara announced, "Mom, I'm going to be a bride!" I'll bet every mother wants to give her daughter a fairy-tale wedding and

I was no exception. But, I wanted it for my Barbara in spades!

She has a learning disability, which prevented her from enjoying a typical childhood. Kids are cruel. They often snubbed her and hurt her feelings, so her early years had been lonely ones. I hoped a beautiful wedding would make up for some of that pain.

Barbara had been so brave, beating all the odds. When she was still in junior high, the doctors told us, "She won't be able to graduate high school. It will be too tough for her. To make it easier, enroll her in private school." When the time came to send her to the special school, she pleaded with me, "Please let me continue in public school. I know I can do it." AND SHE DID! She not only graduated from high school, but, later, earned her BA degree. Now, she's a physical therapy assistant and works with the geriatric population. *It's so typical of my Barbara to want to help those who can't help themselves.*

Now, she had met her "*Doctor Charming*" and was making wedding plans. *Imagine, my first born engaged to a wonderful boy who was in medical school. That's every mother's dream and it was coming true for me!* Surely, it doesn't get any better than that!

We immediately got busy looking for a place to have the wedding, and taking care of other delightful details like flowers, music, photographers, and invitations. However, my main focus...dresses!

In mid-November, I scored! While just browsing with my friend, Esther, I accidentally stumbled across the perfect dress...the right color, the right style, and on sale...absolutely perfect! Well, *almost perfect...*

It didn't exactly fit me. It was a few inches too small to zip up. Immediately, the dressmaker was summoned, "Let's

34

make a deal," she said. "I can let it out a bit, and you could lose a few pounds." No problem! A piece of cake (*pardon the expression*). After all, the wedding was not until March and it was only November.

Abruptly, I stopped humming along with Barbra Streisand. Once again, I could feel the pain of those months. All of December, January and February, I promised myself every morning, "This is the day, I will stay on my diet." Every night, I went to bed hating myself for breaking that promise.

I tried a different diet every single day. *After all, I had dozens at my disposal, pulled from the vast arsenal I had gathered in my lifetime...but nothing was working!*

Being the lady I am, I cannot repeat the names I called myself. The disgust I felt at my inability to stick to a simple diet was robbing me of my joy. *Damn it, FAT, you are spoiling the excitement of my daughter's wedding.*

I did find an eleventh hour reprieve, however. For the three weeks before the wedding, I was on a complete liquid fast. *It was no fun, but I figured, I earned it...and I got it!*

The wedding was magnificent...one of the most wonderful nights of my life. My daughter looked like a fairy-tale princess as she glided down the aisle in her beautiful wedding gown to marry her tall and handsome prince. Looking around at all my dear ones, my eyes filled with tears. I felt like the luckiest person alive...a loving partner at my side, beautiful children, a warm and caring family, and terrific friends. No way it gets any better than that! *Howard also had tears in his eyes. He was thinking about how much all of this was costing and trying to figure out exactly where to get the money to pay for it.*

What an evening! Everything was divine. The flowers were gorgeous...the music terrific...the food was getting rave reviews... and the dessert table looked magnificent.

I was having such a marvelous time, that even the fasting seemed worthwhile. Pity, it didn't last! Just as we were about to leave...DISASTER! The seam of my elegant new dress split!

Congratulations, FAT, you scored another victory. Looks like you have always won. Barbra, I'm so sorry, but I have no happy days to report.

As the song ended, we pulled into the mall parking lot and headed for the food court. With a silent thanks to Barbra Streisand, I walked up to the pizza counter and ordered, "One slice of pizza and a diet soda, please." Then, I congratulated myself for being smart enough to include a provision in my original THIN LIFESTYLE to control myself at a food court. Pizza and a drink, my pre-determined choice, designed to help me avoid temptation when I was struggling. Boy, I had been in trouble, this day, and had almost blown it BIG TIME. Fortunately, my THIN LIFE-STYLE was there to help me.

Forget it, FAT, this is one happy day that belongs to me...not you!

On the way home, I was elated. Unquestionably, I had triumphed, but I made a vow never to forget the pain of being out of control. I needed it to remind me that I never wanted to return to a time when I was a slave to food. No binge is worth my self-respect. Besides, I didn't need a temporary solution to handle my problems. I didn't want to build a wall of food to keep out pain because that very same wall also keeps out joy.

I knew I had to cut my emotional ties to food, but that is some tall order. I found out just how "tall" when Steve was home from college for the summer.

It's always delightful to have my son home, in spite of the mess he makes. He's so much fun, and whenever he's there, our house is filled with activity! *For sure, I always know the daily "up to the minute" baseball scores whenever he's around.*

As the summer drew to an end, I began dreading the day Steve would leave. The house would seem so empty without him and this time it was no "ordinary departure." Steve had already announced that since he was in the last year of his MBA, he wanted a place of my own, and wouldn't be coming home to live after graduation. Hey, wait a minute! That's not fair! He's <u>my baby</u>! *Who said he could grow up, anyway? I certainly didn't remember giving my permission!*

To make matters worse, this year I couldn't go up to Gainesville to help him set up his apartment. *He might be an honors student, but totally incompetent to deal with hanging pictures, putting up shelves and arranging furniture.* As usual, I was recovering from surgery, so the only logical option...send Howard.

The guys planned to get an early start on the morning of their departure and while I'm not now—nor have I ever been—a morning person, I did want to wish them a happy trip. So, I got up and hustled downstairs for the big "bon voyage." To play it for the full effect, I even stood in the doorway waving goodbye. I figured they would never know that I'd be back in bed and sound asleep before they reached the end of our street.

Alone at last! Time to go back to bed and sleep 'til noon. As I started up the stairs, I was stricken with an overwhelming urge to eat Oreo cookies. From the top of my head to the tip of my toes, I craved those cookies. And since its my nature to always have a little something put aside for "emergencies," I knew just where I had tucked away an unopened package of Oreos. As I started to get them, I was overcome by a couple of very strange thoughts. *"Why do I want to eat at this ungodly time of the morning? And, there's no way in hell I want to eat ONE lousy Oreo."*

I wanted to eat and eat and EAT. In fact, I doubted there were enough cookies on the face of the earth to satisfy me at that moment. I needed those cookies...or did I? What did I need? What was I feeling? One thing for sure, it wasn't hunger!

The last of my tribe was leaving. My baby had grown up, and the possibility existed, he would soon find a girl and get married.

Hysterically, I told myself, "I bet she'll hate me. I KNOW she will, and she'll never let him be <u>my baby</u> again. Who was SHE, anyway, to tell me that SHE'D take care of him from now on?" I hate HER...whoever SHE is! Damn it, I never should have permitted this to happen. How did my baby get from Oreos to girls so fast anyway? This must be my fault. There had to be some way I could have prevented this from happening.

Then, it hit me! I didn't want a cookie! I wanted to give my baby a cookie...one more time. I wanted my mother to give me a cookie, and one of her warm and wonderful hugs, that always assured me that everything was going to be all right.

Come on Oreos! Do your magic. Can't you see I'm hurting? Wait a minute! What magic?

My baby has grown up and I have to face it. He isn't coming back and eating Oreos can't change that. I'll have to find another way to comfort myself...without the cookies...and without the hug. I thought it over for a moment. Why am I here alone with my baby on the way to a life of his own? It was simple! I didn't have enough children! But, that wasn't my fault. I wanted more children. It was Howard who hadn't wanted more than three. Clearly, as usual, my suffering was his fault! If he had let me have more children,

Steve wouldn't be the baby, and I wouldn't be facing the *empty nest syndrome*...NOW.

Instantly, that revelation made me feel better, so I didn't need the cookies. Instead, I did what any normal THIN woman would have done in that situation. I had a good cry and went back to bed. After all, it was only 8:30 in the morning...and none of the major department stores were open yet!

CHAPTER
7

AN ATTITUDE ADJUSTMENT

During the next several months, I discovered there is a fine line between success and failure. In the rigid world of dieting, I failed over and over because diets require perfection, and measure success only in pounds. I demand a new yardstick! First, please remove the words **perfect** and **failure** from my vocabulary...

Perfect is much too much trouble to fool with...and far too heavy to carry around. Besides, it's a relief to admit to making an occasional mistake. And failure? Exactly what is it anyway? When does it happen? When do you fail? How long do you get before the jury comes in with a verdict?

Is trying something new—that doesn't work—a failure? In the DIET WORLD, there was no provision for "trial and error" so, I didn't know much about it. They branded me a cheater the minute I committed the first small indiscretion. If I cheated, I blew it... and if I blew it...I QUIT.

I can't believe that I ever accepted the philosophy of the DIET WORLD because my personal philosophy is so different. For an "attitude adjustment," I went to a logical source for guidance...my memory.

Janet, my middle child, was always afraid of failure, hesitant to throw "caution to the wind" and take chances. (*She certainly did not inherit that trait from me. It must have been from someone on Howard's side.*)

When the time came to think about college, she grew leery. "I'm just not ready for a sleep-away experience," she said, "so I think I will take some courses at a local junior college." *I'm no fool. I was tired of dealing with her messy room and figured it was time for a serious talk about her future.* "Janet dear, what do you plan to do with your life?" She quickly announced, "I want to be president of IBM."

Gently I mentioned the likelihood that perhaps she might require a good college education to reach that lofty goal. Then, I made her an offer I was hoping she could not refuse, "Go to the University of Florida and just try it! If you don't like it...no harm done. You can come home and attend any local school of your choice." She agreed...and off she went.

She loved it! She became "little sister" to a fraternity and studied amazingly hard. (*So hard in fact, I heard they have retired her seat in the UF library, since she spent so much time in it.*)

Before we knew it, she graduated with the highest of honors. She tried...and she made it! She had taken a chance and scored a huge success. To my amazement, she even decided to go for her MBA and, immediately, began sending for graduate school literature.

After careful study, she chose to go to a southern school. I didn't think that was a super idea, so I cautioned her, "Juj, you are an *Easterner*. You will have nothing in common with the *southern* girls and may not be very happy there." *Of course, she ignored my counsel and decided to go anyway. Since SHE was the college graduate, who was I to argue with her?*

She *flew* out to school for an early orientation. *No dummy, my kid! It was Howie and I who inherited the job of driving the U-Haul, with all her worldly possessions, from Florida to Louisiana.* We did all we could to help her get settled, however, I was very nervous. I hated the thought of leaving her there, fearing that she wouldn't be comfortable. *My poor child! There wasn't even a Bloomingdale's in town.*

When the time came for me to leave, I crossed my fingers, wished for the best, and went home. Six weeks later she called crying, "I'm totally miserable. I hate it here. My life is over." Realizing how difficult it was for her to admit that she had made a serious mistake, I caught the first plane to Louisiana to bring her home...*in disgrace!*

On the long car trip home, I expounded my personal philosophy, A MISTAKE IS NOT A FAILURE. A mistake is just something that goes wrong and...you fix it! *Why else would they put erasers on pencils?*

I urged her to try again, "There are many universities in the east that will be more than willing to give you a chance to earn your MBA. All that is necessary is that you're willing to continue. Your dream isn't gone, Janet, it has just suffered a temporary delay." It wasn't easy to convince her, but I did! She went back to school—and after earning her MBA—got a fabulous job. *She may not be the president yet; but, she's on her way! You guessed it! She works for IBM!*

Her experience reminded me that only by following your dream can you find the path to making it a reality. It worked for my Janet and it is going to work for me. I am going to follow my dream until I make it come true. My philosophy of life can be my philosophy for getting to my ideal weight...YOU NEVER FAIL UNTIL YOU STOP TRYING.

CHAPTER
8

THE THIN WEIGH IS BORN

My confidence grew. I found myself handling many areas of my life I had never been able to handle before. Making my own choices, my new attitude, and all that I had discovered made me proud. It also convinced me that for most of my life, I had believed a lie. I hated the pain I had endured and loathed the fact that others were still suffering. I detested the ads I saw in newspapers, promising FAST, EASY and PERMANENT weight losses, and wished I could forbid them.

How can a weight loss be **permanent** if it only confronts food, and food is not the issue? Merely losing weight is not enough—the weight will simply be regained—if the true issues of obesity are not being addressed.

I yearned to shout the truth from the roof tops, "It's not our fault. We didn't fail...the DIET WORLD did." I wanted to assure others, "You can be free from the lifelong curse of dieting and overeating which leads only to misery and failure."

Again, it was fate that was kind...it brought me Judy. As part of my campaign to love myself, I decided to treat myself to long, glorious fingernails. For some reason, I didn't seem to be able to grow them, so I opted for the acrylics.

I remembered that my former diet club lecturer owned a nail salon. I hadn't seen her for quite some time because I dropped out of her class to do my own thing. I missed her, and this was a terrific opportunity to "kill two birds with one stone," so I immediately called for an appointment.

In the weeks and months that followed, while Judy made my hands gorgeous, we talked about food—about dieting—and about control. We both had shared the problems of being overweight, but not in the same way...or for the same reasons.

Since she was the most dynamic and motivating lecturer on the face of the earth, I never recognized that she, too, struggled with the rigid concepts of dieting. I benefitted greatly from her eighteen years of experience and truly respected her opinion. With her input and support, I felt no qualms about bringing forth our new attitude. Together, Judy and I gave birth to THE THIN WEIGH!

With the help of Eileen Cypress, M.D., we developed a simple plan...THE THIN WEIGH LIFESTYLER...designed to teach dieters how to choose any food, without guilt, and in control. Dr. Cypress was responsible for recommending the minimum daily requirements of each food group to insure proper nourishment for the body. Within the groups, however, there is freedom of choice and, best of all, no foods are "forbidden!" Ours is a plan for life and does not demand that anyone give up the foods they love...FOREVER!

Now, I needed a forum; a way to share this valuable information and so THE THIN WEIGH, a "food control organization," was incorporated. Its sole mission was to find a way to put itself out of business. I prayed that someday it would not be necessary for anyone ever to need what I had to offer. My hope was that my new message would make dieting obsolete.

When the announcement of the birth of THE THIN WEIGH appeared in the *Miami Herald*, panic gripped me. In fact, I was almost paralyzed with fear. What if no one came? Or what if someone came, but I wasn't able to make them understand...or believe me? What if I wasn't good enough? Or what if no one wanted my new philosophy? What if...indeed?

What if...what I had to say helped someone else the way it had helped me? To help others end their pain would be worth anything I had to endure.

Luckily, people came. On a rainy Thursday night I gave my first lecture to what later became "a small band of loyal followers." THE THIN WEIGH had made a firm beginning...and I was overjoyed!

I began to share my new attitude, my experiences, my THIN LIFESTYLE and, to my delight, others began to accept my new concept. Together, we were all fighting for control, learning from each other, and best of all...losing weight.

What's more, we were achieving our heart's desire and becoming what we had always dreamed we could be. Look out, DIET WORLD, with any luck, your day's are numbered!

The concept that began in my mind during the sleepless night, when I took the responsibility for my FAT, now had a name...THE THIN WEIGH. Imagine that! What started as a "maybe" is now a force to be reckoned with.

Never again can the DIET WORLD fool us! We were proving that anybody can be THIN. It takes no special talent, just DETERMINATION, MOTIVATION, and the right INFORMATION.

PART

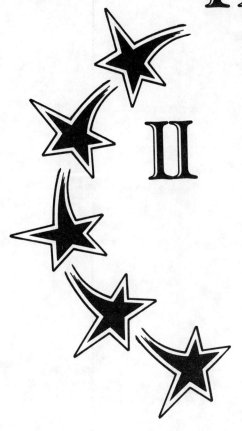

II

JOURNEY
TO
FREEDOM

CHAPTER 9

A NEW FRONTIER

I DID IT! I made the successful transition...I am a THIN person. As a reward, I have earned the opportunity to guide my members from the DIET WORLD...to the THIN WORLD! Imagine me, a tour director! Of course, taking such a fabulous trip sounded glorious, but, nevertheless, the awesome responsibility I had undertaken absolutely terrified me. Believe it or not, it was my job to lead my people out of bondage to a new frontier—sort of like a blend of Moses and Neil Armstrong...

So what...if my small band of THIN WEIGH pioneers was "just a drop in the bucket" to what we needed to wipe out the DIET WORLD? I was still very proud of them for having the foresight to see the future...and the courage to step into it.

For as long as I can remember, I had always been a science fiction nut, so seeking a new frontier was right up my alley! Back in the '50's, I saw the movie, *Destination Moon*, a dozen or more times. During that film, I remember watching in awe as a rocket landed on the moon, a man got out, walked on the surface, and planted the American flag.

Back then, it boggled the imagination! I never believed

THAT could happen in my lifetime—and yet—in my lifetime ...IT happened! I still get "goose bumps" thinking about Neil Armstrong taking "one giant step for mankind" by setting foot on the moon. Now, I had the chance to take a "giant step" of my own.

My little group was truly ahead of its time, and, accordingly, we were a bit apprehensive. It's scary to leave home and hearth—pull up stakes—and go exploring the unknown. I speculated that, perhaps, if we took a look at the past, it would make it easier to picture the future.

Let's try to imagine what life was like in Dodge City in the 1800's. Were the folks of the Old West ONLY contented with their lot because they had no knowledge that life could be easier? I think so! For sure that's the ONLY reason I remained in the world of diets. What choice did I have? It was the ONLY world I could perceive—the ONLY world that existed for me—the ONLY world for a FAT person. Sure, it was strict, but I didn't know any better.

Do you think if we gave the residents of those days a glimpse of our modern day world, we could persuade them to relocate? I'm betting that they would jump at the chance for a better life after enduring a lifetime of hardship. Remember Dodge City didn't have even the simplest form of luxuries...the ones we just take for granted. Let's take a look at yesterday's world...

In Dodge City, the Medicine Man was always a welcome sight when he rode into town. As the people gathered around his colorfully painted wagon, the cunning con man tried to persuade them he had a magic elixir...to cure whatever ailed them. Looking back NOW from our vantage point, we chuckle at the thought the people of his day actually believed his elixir had magical healing powers. Sure, we can laugh. In hindsight, it's easy to see it for exactly

48

what it was...just a hoax...snake oil!

The clever Medicine Man made the same elixir in different colors—so he could use the same product—which cured nothing—as a cure for everything. From the side of his wagon, he bellowed, "Hurry, hurry, hurry, come and get it! My magic elixir can cure anything. Take your pick: red...for fever, blue...for arthritis, yellow...for pneumonia, green...for tonsillitis."

The smooth-talking, charismatic swindler concentrated on the gullible and ignored the hecklers. "Forget the failures of the past. They are not applicable. This elixir is NEW AND IMPROVED...absolutely guaranteed to work."

I can't blame these people of yesteryear for being gullible ...so was I. Every Sunday, I scanned the newspaper looking for ads that promised "FAST and EASY" weight losses. Tell me, what's the difference between today's "miracle diets" and yesterday's "magic elixirs?" Not much! NEW and IMPROVED diets are constantly appearing—ignoring all past failures—absolutely guaranteed to work.

Our modern day Medicine Man bellows, "Hurry, hurry, hurry, come and get it. Take your pick: all protein, all carbohydrates, pills, shots, wraps...or packaged foods."

Baloney! Trying to cure obesity with diets is like trying to cure it with...snake oil.

At last, after years of hawking bizarre food combinations, all claiming to be "fat burning, chemically balanced, scientific approaches to weight loss"...PROGRESS! A new breed of Medicine Man rode into town offering the ultimate solution —the cure of cures—NO FOOD AT ALL! Remarkably, we had come full circle! Once again, we gathered around to listen to a fast-talking con man offering magical, brightly colored, liquid elixirs. "Hurry, hurry, hurry, come and get it. Take your pick: Liquid Protein, Cambridge, Herbalife, or

Opti-Fast."

I bought it all...hook, line and sinker! Faithfully, I divided my veggies into categories: Group One...eaten only in the daytime and Group Two...eaten only at night. I never demanded to know how my stomach knew the difference. *I didn't ask my doctor, "Does my stomach have a clock or a calendar in it? If so, how come you never detected one with X-rays, sonograms, or the like?"*

Foolishly without protesting, I followed the dictates of diets that alleged to work only on Monday, Tuesday or Wednesday. *How silly! Why didn't I ask, "What will happen if I try them on Thursday, Friday or Saturday? Will I gain weight?"*

I didn't ask HOW or WHY because I didn't want to know. I followed instructions because in the final analysis, I was a coward! I was afraid I'd have "no control" without a step-by-step program...and didn't believe that I could lose weight without dieting. Hoping that any moment the **perfect** diet would materialize and provide a "quick-fix" suited me better then facing the difficult task of finding a way to control myself. But, I paid a high price. Life in the DIET WORLD was harsh...absent of the luxuries of choice, pride, and freedom.

No more! Now—a new truth—DIETS NEVER WORK. So, let's fire up our rockets. Good-bye yesterday, we have set our sights on a new frontier—a place where we can live with peace of mind and never again have to agonize about our weight—our destination: THIN!

CHAPTER
10

TRAVELLING LIGHT

Thank heavens, I'm so smart. I had the good sense to know it would be useless to haul "FAST...EASY...AND... EXCITING" on our journey to THIN. We'd be travelling light and didn't need the burden of these unrealistic expectations. Sure, it would be painful to sort through the diet memories of a lifetime. But, it had to be done in order for us to discard our cumbersome excess baggage. To make it easier to let go of our diet legacy, I racked my brain for brilliant examples of how these cruel myths had never helped us in the past. *Seek and ye shall find...*

One night right after New Year's, as I was coming out of a diet food store (savoring an ice cream cone), I encountered Rosalie and Paulina in the parking lot. Instinctively, I knew they were coming from a diet club meeting. *I guess twenty years of personal experience allowed me to recognize that "January look." I could picture the imaginary shopping bag they were carrying to stock up on all the "diet stuff" they needed for the after-the-holidays-start-up.*

Although they both knew of my involvement with THIN WEIGH, for some reason, it didn't stop Rosalie from saying, "We're just coming from our diet club meeting." *Thanks a heap for that wonderful news. Sure, give your money to the competition...then ask for my blessings.*

In reply, Howie almost caused me to die of embarrassment when he stated point blank, "You're wasting your money on your group...switch programs immediately! Suzie is a marvelous lecturer and all her members love her." *Suddenly, my embarrassment turned to pride. I congratulated myself for selecting such a perceptive man as a husband.*

I've always believed "if it ain't broke—don't fix it," so I contradicted Howie by saying, "Rosalie and Paulina, it's best for you to continue with your own program. Unless, of course, it isn't helping you." Quite indignantly, Rosalie snapped back, "My program **ALWAYS** works for me. I lost FIFTY-THREE pounds last year.

For the life of me, I couldn't figure out WHY she said that. *She didn't look even a pound thinner then the last time I saw her.* I kid you not, this girl easily had fifty or sixty pounds to lose and it would shock me if **any** program came forward to claim the credit for her success.

Frankly, I didn't know exactly what to say, so I began fishing for just the right words. I knew this situation deserved extreme caution. I still remembered how much it hurt me when someone greeted me by saying, "Boy, you look like you really gained a lot of weight." *I've often wondered what people were thinking when they were so rude. Maybe, they figured I hadn't noticed? Or did they think it was possible I had confused the clothes hanging in my closet...which didn't fit me anymore...with those accidentally left behind by a band of traveling gypsies? Or maybe, they expected me to thank them for reminding me of my pain.*

No matter, to play it smart with Rosalie, I just kept listening. She rationalized, "Every January, I go to my diet club—avoid all bad foods—and lose fifty quick pounds. When I've had it with the deprivation—and can no longer endure it—I binge eat—and find the fifty pounds again. Then, every January, I go back to my diet club."

Honestly, with all her heart, she believes her program ALWAYS works for her. Of course, she's overlooking the obvious. What she considers **ALWAYS** is—in fact—**NEVER!** A quick weight loss—a quicker weight gain—NEVER allows her to be a THIN person. She stays a perpetual dieter... forever!

Henceforth, we will be cheering for the tortoise and not betting on the hare!

Now, we had to deal with the expectation that every meal should be a gastronomical experience. Imagine having the job of planning menus that are thrilling, stimulating, and delicious...three   meals a day...seven days a week. Sounds like quite a challenge, especially when food was intended to be the "staff of life"...not the "spice of life."

Where in the world did we get the notion that every meal has to be inspiring? *Do you think it was from Lynn Redgrave? A hundred times a day on television, she yanks off her clothes and shrieks, "This is living." Gads, we are in trouble if our only way to true happiness is to consume a variety of exciting frozen foods.*

Let's face it, life can't always be *spicy*. Unfortunately, much of our time must be spent doing the "nitty gritty." Every morning, when I wake up, I take a shower and brush my teeth. For as long as I can remember, I head for the hairdresser every Friday. Am I bored with my routine? I wouldn't rule out the possibility that I am, but so what? I never give it any thought. Why should I? Even bored, I'm never going to stop showering and brushing my teeth. And, I wouldn't advise you to hold your breathe waiting for me to ask my hairdresser, "Richie, how much longer do I have to come here?" *Actually, he's not boring...he's a doll...but what's the difference? He does magic with my hair and that's what really counts!*

In that same regard, even if I don't find euphoria in every meal I eat, I'm not going to give up my THIN LIFESTYLE. For the rest of my life, it's my job to take care of myself... including the simple function of eating! But, that's me! Not everyone feels that way.

One morning, one of my regular, long-standing members called me. "I'm not planning to continue coming to class," she said. "Why, Carol" I asked, "why are you leaving when you are doing so well?" Her response briefly cheered me, "I love the program. It gives me more flexibility and freedom than any other I've ever tried. Being able to make my own choices is fantastic and I enjoy the fact that no foods are "forbidden."

Sounded good to me. "So, what's the problem, Carol? Why don't you stay?" Sadly she replied, "I'm sorry, I just can't. I'm bored." Then sensing my disappointment, she continued, "Suzie, it's not you...you are the best lecturer I've ever heard. Your presentations are creative and your classes are fun." *(Thanks, I needed that! When someone quits, I plague myself with doubts. Was there anything I could have done to keep them? Maybe, if I had been a bit more motivating...if I had explained our new attitude just a little better... if I had been stronger or weaker...or what...maybe, they would have stayed.)*

Bottom line for Carol—her food was boring! *Of course, she didn't find her fifty-eight pound weight loss too shabby!* However, binge eating was her favorite form of excitement, and in light of her boredom, she didn't feel she could continue.

Talking to her was like "*deja vu*," as I just had a similar conversation with my son. He was six months away from completing his MBA, but complained, "Mom, school is very boring. For the last five and half years, I've been stuck in a very small town. Not only that, but the work I'm doing is a repeat of what I studied in undergraduate school...and I'm not a bit stimulated. I want to come home."

"Steven, of course, you <u>must</u> come home immediately! It would be unreasonable to expect you to stay in Gainesville for six more months...if you're bored. Please disregard all the years you have already invested. Who cares if you forfeit your MBA? My son, if excitement is your top priority—and your MBA pales in comparison—I fully agree that you have but one alternative...pick excitement."

And that's exactly what I offered Carol! Pick more exciting eating...or pick THIN. I went 50–50. My son stayed...Carol left.

Naturally, I hate to see anyone succumb to the EASY way —yet, I had to face that its appeal is often too strong to overcome. One night, beautiful Kerry joined one of my classes. She was barely thirteen years old, but already an expert on dieting. No matter how obscure the food, she could tell me the exact number of calories it had. However, she had a deeply entrenched "diet mentality" and was only looking for a QUICK and EASY way to lose weight. Over the next several weeks, she constantly whined, "It's awfully tough to eat a little bit of something I like. It's very difficult to stop eating when I want more." *(I can't imagine what made her think __THAT__ was news to me!)*

Her honesty was refreshing, though. She made no bones about the fact that she wasn't looking for a tough job. Therefore, I wasn't a bit surprised when she finally told me straight out, "I don't think THIN WEIGH is for me. There are just too many choices. I'd rather not have to face the enemy every day." Obviously I hated to lose her, but I did

...to a *liquid* diet. *I know she will return someday. I doubt she can avoid food for the rest of her life and, for sure, food won't go away. To find peace, she will have to conquer it!*

Gosh, I wish I did know an EASY way to change the habits of a lifetime. Wouldn't it be lovely if reprogramming a FAT brain was EASY? Sorry, Kerry, it's not. You are fighting a formidable enemy...FOOD. Besides, perpetuating the illusion there is an EASY way to lose weight leads to denial, dishonesty, and defeat.

The real truth is that dismantling the "diet mentality" and accepting the fact that there are no magic formulas...magic elixirs...or magic wands...IS difficult. But, it's the truth—and armed with the truth—we will have the power to win—for the truth will set us free.

CHAPTER
11

HOW ARE WE GONNA GET THERE?

Helping so many different people lose weight is quite a challenge...except for the DIET WORLD. They still insist that <u>ONE</u> diet will work for everyone. Ridiculous! How can one diet meet the needs of so many different people? It can't! Obviously, that's why there are so few successful dieters. And, of course, while they promise that if you follow their plan your weight will simply "melt off," they neglect to mention the deprivation, starvation, and humiliation that you'll encounter along the way...

Sure reaching the destination is important, but so is enjoying the trip. That's why our journey is personalized... no rigid timetables, no rules and regulations, no pre-planned itinerary. Everyone can chart their own course.

I hate to fly. I absolutely dread it! Whenever we travel, I'm always politicking to go by car. It's a pity, but I just can't look forward to an excursion that involves an airplane. Not only do I complain constantly about how much I hate to fly, I feel cheated out of the pleasure of making the trip. I feel exactly the same way about a diet! I dread the dieting so much that it diminishes my enthusiasm at the prospect of losing weight. And with that attitude, of course, I'm defeated before I begin.

I do love a car trip...no mail, no telephones, no errands to run, *no praying your plane doesn't hit the side of a mountain* ...just pure relaxation.

However, I'd never taken a car trip ALONE until a call came from Gainesville that one of our kids needed help...and it was urgent. *I don't remember the exact nature of the emergency, but it was probably something expensive. ALL emergencies involving our kids were expensive!*

And talk about quick thinking, Howard immediately became intensely involved in the "audit of a lifetime" and couldn't possibly get away for the world's most boring ride—the Florida Turnpike. I was the one! I was needed! At first I was a little apprehensive about taking a six hour trip alone, but I'm a grown woman with a valid driver's license. No problem, I can do it. *At least, that's what everyone who didn't want to go assured me.* Since this would be a great credit to my name in "Mother of the Year" competition, I decided to go.

At the "crack of dawn" *(dawn does "crack" at 9:00 A.M., right?)*—I threw my little bag in the trunk, buckled up, and departed. The minute I turned my key in the ignition...I WAS IN HEAVEN. I WAS ALONE! No one to tell me WHAT TO DO...or HOW TO DO IT!

Defiantly, just to spite my kids, I set the radio to the "elevator music" station, even though, I don't like that kind of music very much. I'll show them! After all, they never permit me to choose the radio station when we're together. It didn't take me too long to get that out of my system. *Sorry Guy Lombardo, you're not for me*! Instead, I plugged in one of my favorite cassettes, bracing myself for choruses of, "I don't like Billy Joel, I don't like Barry Manilow, I don't like Barbra Streisand." Wonderously, there was not a sound in the car. *Know what? Silence is not golden...it's glorious!*

The trip was going so well, I even started singing along with the tape. *In all honesty, I can't sing. Truly, I have to admit, I have a voice like a sick frog. However, with no one there to remind me how badly I sing, I heard a strong resemblance between my voice and that of Beverly Sills.*

You know it's really true, time does fly when you're having fun...ALONE. Soon I made my way to the first rest stop on the turnpike. Singing along at the top of my lungs dried me up and I needed a break. A devilish thought crossed my mind, "It's my trip, so I am going to stop at EVERY plaza ...whether I need to or not." Howard and the kids would go MAD if they were with me. They always made me feel that it was a "fatal flaw" to require use of the facilities more than most. We always fought in the car because I <u>needed</u> to stop and they <u>didn't</u>. *(It always seemed odd to me that a husband, wife, and three of their own biological children, couldn't coordinate use of the facilities any better than we did.)*

Six hours later I arrived in Gainesville...euphoric! My first solo trip had been a wonderful experience. I loved charting my own course, traveling at my own speed, stopping as many times as I wanted to, and still arriving happily at my destination.

AT LAST! I FINALLY FOUND THE MAP TO DESTINATION THIN! SINCE OURS IS A TRIP TO FREEDOM...A SPECIAL BILL OF RIGHTS...WILL LEAD OUR WAY.

CHAPTER
12

MASTER OF MY FATE

THE THIN BILL OF RIGHTS

WE THE PEOPLE admit that diets cannot make us THIN. Therefore, we are willing and able to take the responsibility for ourselves...resolve our own problems with solutions that suit our needs...forgive ourselves for our past mistakes...identify and deal with our feelings...accept ourselves with our strengths and with our weaknesses...take risks and measure results. WE know the pursuit of our happiness belongs to us...and only to us. WE know the power is within ourselves to get what we need...what we want...and what we are entitled to...

I. I'M ENTITLED TO CHANGE

The past can be a lesson for the future as we can learn much from it. For too long I stubbornly held on to the perception that dieting would make me THIN. Sure, I was suckered in by losing weight; yet, I ignored the fact that the weight loss was like a boomerang...it kept returning. Dieting brought me agony...heartache...and misery, but I accepted it because it allowed me to retain some sense of my own integrity. The diet became my scapegoat!

DIETS ARE MERELY MENTAL CUL-DE-SACS! Consequently, I became trapped in a vicious cycle that blocked the development of the necessary problem solving skills I needed to escape. Instead, the lessons I learned from dieting strengthened my negative attitude and reinforced my feelings of helplessness.

Liquid diets taught me I couldn't starve. I wanted food. The doctor's cookie diet taught me I preferred Oreos. Diet classes taught me I couldn't consistently live with a plan that was inconsistent to my values as it forced me to cheat and feel guilty.

Luckily, fate always came to my rescue. When I moved from one end of the city to another and was desperate to make new friends, I met Ellen...a naturally THIN person. *I was lonely and she was very kind to me or I probably would have waited for a FAT friend to come along.* Thank goodness I'm not patient for it was my friendship with Ellen that helped me uncover some of the basic differences between being FAT and being THIN.

No size 22½ looks forward to "breaking bread" with a size 8 and, naturally, I didn't want her to think I was FAT because I ate too much. *I wanted her to think I had a severe glandular condition!* So, whenever we went out to eat together, I cautiously allowed her to order first. I figured if I ate whatever she ate, my secret would be safe.

One day at lunch, she ordered a tuna fish sandwich on white toast with lettuce. *Not so bad, I could always eat something else when I got home if that wasn't enough for me ...so I ordered the same.* When the waiter brought our lunch

61

to the table, she exclaimed, "My word, what a big sandwich! I could never eat ALL THAT FOOD." I looked down at my identical portion and pondered, "Where? Where is ALL THAT FOOD she's talking about?" *Then I wondered, "If she really can't finish her lunch, what are the chances I could get her leftovers...without her seeing me?"*

Did Ellen's body need less food than mine? Was her stomach any smaller than my stomach? Nope! It was all coming from the brain. She thought...THIN! I thought... FAT!

Excuse me IBM, but you know it's the human brain that functions as the world's most sophisticated computer. The only problem is that it simply cannot tell the difference between right and wrong. It believes whatever you tell it— or allow anyone else to tell it—thereby allowing perception to function as truth.

The best a diet could do was make me temporarily food free. Trouble is, I stayed a FAT person trying to resist food, and there is much, much more to becoming a THIN person, then simply resisting food. Changing FAT software to the mind-set of a THIN person is a <u>must</u>. For sure, a major reprogramming was in order for me, like the one I had when I stopped smoking.

For the first year after I quit, I behaved like a "smoker" trying to resist cigarettes. Gradually as time passed, I became more and more comfortable with not smoking. Eventually I became a "non-smoker"...and have been for the last twelve years. Now, envisioning myself walking over to an ash tray —shuffling through it until I located the best looking butt— straightening up that little sucker and lighting it—because I was out of cigarettes—is hardly one of my fondest memories. Disgusting! But, no more disgusting then binge eating.

Reprogramming means making a commitment to a new way

of life...a THIN life. At first, treating myself as a THIN person was a bit awkward. *I realize many servers behind a buffet line had a good chuckle when I asked for a small portion of something. I explained, "I am a very small eater." I'm sure they thought, "Ha, ha, ha, size 22½..a small eater! A small cow...or what?"* So what? It didn't matter one bit what they thought. Only what my brain believed was important.

What a dunce! I can't imagine why it took me so long to figure that out? Suddenly the years I spent in the FAT WORLD seemed kind of silly. After all, dieting to become THIN makes about as much sense, as studying the work of Babe Ruth, if your goal is to play quarterback for the Miami Dolphins.

Let's face it, I had no reason to hang on to even a glimmer of hope that the perfect diet was just a heartbeat away...or that wishing would one day make me THIN. Besides, I didn't need that kind of stuff anymore. I knew it was my image of myself that would determine what I would become. THIN was within me. The power to change was mine! For years I had waited—just hoping it would happen—now I was going to make it happen!

All I needed to be THIN was the commitment to change. Enough "would have"..."could have"...or "should have." Goodbye "what if"...or "how come." So long to diets...excuses...guilt ...and self-recrimination. From this day forward, I will THINK like a THIN person...I will ACT like a THIN person ...I will EAT like a THIN person...and I will BECOME a THIN person.

II. I'M ENTITLED TO MAKE MY OWN CHOICES

The DIET WORLD denied me the privilege of making my own choices. I had to be strict, strict, strict. No deviations, no cheating, no exceptions...*no time off for good behavior.* "Follow your diet <u>precisely</u> or you won't lose weight." Denying me my right to self-determination stripped me of my dignity and forced me to become a master manipulator...

THIN people never doubt their intelligence—question their ability—or their right to make their own choices. But me? The DIET WORLD made it quite clear they didn't trust me! After all, how can you trust a cheater? I had no willpower! I was weak! Certainly, they couldn't allow me to decide for myself what foods would constitute my daily allowance of calories. They treated me like an incompetent imbecile and presumed it was better for them to make ALL my choices for me.

Baloney! Willpower was not my problem. *If I didn't have willpower, then how did I lose over a ton in my lifetime?* It was won't power, I didn't have. I simply didn't want to live the rest of my life by someone else's regulations. Truth is, I don't like anyone to tell me what to do. "Don't eat that." "Lose faster." "Starve yourself." So when they do...I rebel... and do the exact opposite. Know what? Their <u>negative</u> brand of willpower stinks!   I'll show them, they are wrong about me. Forget what I can't or won't do...here's my new <u>positive</u> willpower: I WILL learn to make my own choices. I WILL eat in control. I WILL BE THIN. I WILL! I WILL! I WILL!

Learning how to control my favorite foods gave me some tough times. *Trust me, no one ever had to support my effort not to eat too much of the foods I hated. I swear, I never abused cottage cheese or yogurt. Yuck!*

It was the battle for the right to eat chocolate that raged in me. I wanted it! During my years in diet class, I tortured my lecturer by insisting, "I need a piece of chocolate after dinner. I WANT IT!" Her effort to convince me, otherwise, was a valiant one. She recommended, "Make yourself an interesting salad, so you won't think about the candy. Use as many veggies as you like, but remember...variety is the key." *Alas, the operation was a success...but the patient died.*

After consuming a salad that would fill Yankee Stadium, guess what I wanted? You got it...a piece of chocolate. No way—NOW—I would have just one. If I had to lie for it, sneak for it, cheat for it...I binged it. *A THIN LIFESTYLE gave me the opportunity to skip the salad.*

Trying to eat around the foods I loved NEVER worked. Let's be honest, I was going to eat them. The issue was whether I was going to eat them...**in-control** or **out-of-control.** Giving myself permission to eat them eliminated my need to cheat and guaranteed that no one will ever call me a cheater again! Alas, I came face to face with the realization that what I had always thought was "*cheating on my diet*" —in reality—had been "*cheating on myself.*" I have no need to cheat anymore. I have the responsibility and the right to spend my calories...**MY WAY.**

I'm a better teacher than I am a student. Years earlier, I taught my kids a similar lesson on our first trip to Disney World. Initially, they made me positively crazy wanting me to buy them everything in sight. They felt absolutely no responsibility for how much money they spent...or how they spent it. The next day, I got smart and gave each of them an envelope with spending money. The deal was simple— they could buy anything they wanted—but when the money was gone—that was it. And, boy, it worked! They became very careful about making their choices! Now, I had the same opportunity. I was free to spend my calories **ANY WAY** I wanted to—but when they were gone—that was it.

In comparison to the black and white rigidity of the DIET WORLD, freedom of choice is indescribable. Although, there are no "failure proof" choices, it doesn't matter. Having the courage to take risks—and feeling free to make mistakes—liberated me from the fear of failure. My aim... PROGRESS NOT PERFECTION.

Dumb choices gave me the opportunity to learn how to make more intelligent choices in the future...wise choices gave me encouragement! Every time I won the battle over food, I felt the power shifting...from food...to ME!

I'll bet Howie breathed a sigh of relief when he heard I was taking responsibility for myself. It got him off the hook! All the years I spent dieting, the poor guy was "damned, if you do"—or—"damned, if you don't." We played out two scenarios...and neither one favored him!

If I wanted to be "good" on my diet, I'd ask him to help me resist temptation. Unfortunately, as soon as the waiter put the wonderful hot bread on the table, my resolve would vanish. I'd polish off a few pieces of bread causing Howie to whisper, ever so softly in my ear, "Honey, you wanted to be good."

I blasted him! Then, I proceeded to order my favorite high calorie dinner. *When it was time for dessert, Howie left the table and hid in the men's room.* Of course, all the way home, I reprimanded him for not being forceful enough to stop me from cheating. Damned, if you do!

The next time we went out, when I again solicited his help, he chose not to get into the "line of fire." So, as I ate with wild abandonment, he said nothing. This time, I griped, "It is obvious to me that you don't care enough about me to even help me stick to a simple diet." Damned, if you don't!

"Bad" foods weren't the only cause of crisis. OUT OF CONTROL IS OUT OF CONTROL! Once, I bought a package of muenster cheese...a "good" food...to eat for lunch. I'm not wild about it; yet, I finished off the entire package. Ashamed of myself, I asked for guidance in diet class. "Keep the package of cheese at your neighbor's house and, every day, just go over and get a slice." Sparkling advice! *No wonder, I couldn't win the battle for control. I wasn't even advised to fight...and everytime I surrendered...food won!*

I got no advice or too much advice. Before going out for dinner one evening, our friends, Judith and Harvey, invited Howie and me to come by for a drink. From the moment I entered their family room, it was apparent Judith didn't know exactly what to serve me. Her gorgeous bar was covered with food...cheese and crackers, peanuts, carrot sticks, fruit, and candy. *(Funny no one ever worries about what to serve a THIN person because they know they can eat anything.)*

Since it was only seven o'clock, I wasn't hungry. Usually I don't eat dinner until after eight, so I just sipped a diet soda while we chatted.

Out of the corner of my eye, I was watching my Howie shoveling in one cracker with cheese after the other. *I swear if his cholesterol doesn't kill him...I will!* I gave him one of my icy stares, and he pledged, "This will be my last one." *My timing is amazing, I always manage to catch him on his last one.* Then, he quickly switched to eating carrot sticks and cherries but, of course, he never stopped eating. For years, my Howie has been on the "see food" diet. *When he sees food...he eats it!*

For some unknown reason, everyone loves to tell me about his or her latest fad diet. *What they don't realize is I'd rather go before the firing squad then ever go on another diet.* In an effort to be polite, I patiently listened as Harvey described his great new program:

Day one	. . . .	veggies
Day two	. . . .	bananas
Day three	. . . .	rice
Day four	. . . .	fish
Day five	. . . .	fruit
Over the weekend...*(if you lived)*		anything you wanted

We lingered at home for about an hour and then left to go to an Italian restaurant. By now I was a bit hungry, so I was busy scanning the menu when the waiter brought the garlic sticks to our table. Immediately, all three of my comrades grabbed a bread stick. *What an amazing coincidence, they were all on the "see food" diet.* I decided to pass on the bread in favor of having pasta for dinner. Everyone—but me —ordered an appetizer and quickly devoured it. Instead, I waited patiently for dinner.

When my salad arrived, I briefly reconsidered the bread. *After all, for the last half hour, I had been listening to the trio at my table singing its praises.* After careful deliberation, I decided to hold firm to my original choice since I wanted the pasta more than I wanted bread. *(Sure I could have had a little bit of each, but I opted for more pasta, and no bread.)*

Ultimately the moment I had been waiting for arrived... dinner. The waiter served veal parmigiana to Howie—chicken cacciatore to Judith—veal and peppers to Harvey—and a big plate of pasta to me! When they saw my pasta—as if they rehearsed it—all three of my dinner companions roared in unison, "Are you going to eat ALL that pasta?"

Incredible! Nobody commented when I ignored the cheese and crackers. Not a word had been spoken when I passed on the garlic bread. There were no cries of outrage when I skipped the appetizer. No one even noticed I hadn't ordered wine. Thus far, I had been fully capable of making my own choices. What happened—all of a sudden—to shake their confidence in me? Who cares? My response, "Just watch me!"

Sure, I enjoyed that moment. It's fun making choices when you trust yourself knowing you have the skills to deal effectively with your life. It's exciting to feel in charge of yourself when you have the confidence to be at ease, relaxed, and capable. It's wonderful to no longer need the approval or validation of others. The *inner peace* of self-acceptance brings me MORE happiness than EVERY pound I've EVER lost on EVERY diet I've EVER been on.

I lost more weight after that evening—becoming living proof —that making choices makes you THIN!

III. I'M ENTITLED TO RESPECT MYSELF

Learning self-respect is no easy task for someone who has grown up believing the quest for **perfection** is attainable. In the DIET WORLD, they told me, "Have a **perfect** day...a **perfect** week...a **perfect** life. Be a **perfect** person—with a **perfect** body—just stay on your diet." Fostering the belief that I "should be" or "could be" **perfect** led me to believe that I simply didn't measure up. The feeling of "I'm not good enough" hurled me into the depths of self-loathing, despair, shame, and humiliation...

However, I didn't blame the DIET WORLD...I blamed myself. I berated myself for my lack of **perfection** and didn't tolerate even the smallest imperfection. That's not fair! In the real world, we are not either "perfect or worthless"... "successful or failures!" Hey, cut me a break, nobody's

perfect.

My friend, Julie, is five feet, eleven inches tall in her stocking feet, and she is never in her stocking feet. That dear lady walks around in shoes with heels so high, I doubt I could even **sit** down comfortably in them. She is blond, beautiful, and very fashionable—so whenever I go anywhere with her—I know we will be noticed.

One day we were running errands in a mall together, when we decided to go to the food court for lunch. As predictable as I am about my pizza for lunch, Julie is equally predictable ...a turkey sandwich, with mayo, on white bread. So, we went our separate ways to get our lunch. As we returned to our table, poor Julie tipped over a giant glass of iced tea. It spilled all over everything...even my pizza.

I got busy helping her clean up the mess, but my main concern was to prevent Julie from feeling embarrassed. Immediately, I assured her, "It was just a simple accident. It could have happened to anyone. Don't worry, I love my pizza with iced tea on it. I'll get you another drink. Just sit here and relax. Besides, I'm sure no one saw us." *Sure, 5 ft. 11, blond, beautiful, fashionable...and no one saw us.* I just didn't know what to do to comfort her.

Finally, we got settled and finished our lunch. Then, as we went off to do our errands, I contemplated, "What would I have said to myself if I had spilled the drink...*moron, imbecile, klutz, idiot?*" I would have beaten myself *emotionally black and blue* for making a simple mistake...and name calling hardly leads to a great deal of self-respect.

After our kids left home, it became apparent that we no longer needed a big four bedroom house. Daily, I'd walk through the empty bedrooms and ask Howie, "What happened to the people who used to sleep in these rooms?" The man is not gentle. He pointed out to me, "Suzie, the handwriting is on the wall. The children don't intend to live with us any longer. Barbara and Mark have a place of their own and Janet and Steve are living away at school and won't be back." *Gosh, I hate it when he's right!*

Since I couldn't have my first choice—having my kids come home to live—we decided to sell the house and began making inquiries about finding a realtor.

Everyone we knew had a friend, aunt, uncle, or cousin, who sold houses, so our phone rang off the hook. We got a zillion calls but there was one voice—in particular—that I liked. She sounded so vibrant and friendly and—not only that —she impressed me with what she had to say. So when she suggested we meet to discuss the listing, I quickly agreed. *Is there any way you can tell over the phone that the person you are speaking to is a size four?   Well, there should be!*

From the moment I opened the front door, we clicked! Accordingly, it was an easy decision to give the listing on our house to Celia. Over the next several months, she and I spent a great deal of time together, as Celia not only sold our old house, but helped us buy our new one. I liked her a lot and I knew she liked me, too. Repeatedly, she would say, "Let's *do lunch*—or better yet—get our husbands together and go out for dinner." I always had an excuse for not going —and the excuse was always the same—size 22½ versus size 4. *This woman is not only THIN, but has enough clothes to fill up the dress department of Sak's...and she looks terrific in every outfit she wears.   I was wearing a tent dress!*

Through her persistence, however, we did eventually develop a terrific friendship. Shortly after I lost my weight, I told her how I felt when we first met. When she heard I hadn't wanted to pursue our friendship because I was FAT, she quickly chastised me, "Shame on you for judging yourself so harshly. Did you think all you had to offer was a dress

71

size? Didn't you realize you had so much more than that to give? Couldn't you see how valuable you are? You are witty, charming, warm, and intelligent." *(See why I loved her?)*

But, the truth of the matter is I didn't see any of that, and it doesn't matter who thinks you are valuable, if you don't see the value in yourself.

Then she added, "And, shame on you for judging me so harshly. Did I strike you as the type of woman who would judge a person by what she was wearing?" *I never knew exactly how to tell her that it had crossed my mind...but only just for a second, of course!*

Self-respect is indescribable. It's a friendship you have with yourself—a magical relationship that allows you to love yourself—as much as you love others. It's the most precious gift you can ever give yourself! Self-respect is believing in yourself—knowing you can do something—and backing it up with the hard work it takes to get it done.

I had an opportunity to learn that lesson as a child, but I think I was just too young to understand it. I adored my grandfather. He was my hero—six foot, three in a generation where five foot, nine was tall. Patiently, he often tried to teach me his code of ethics...a hard day's work is the best way to feel good about yourself. Incredibly generous, he would give me just about anything I asked for...but with a string attached. He always asked, "Did you earn it?" *Luckily, he accepted my word, so I said, "Of course, I earned it"*—whether I did or not!

A diet is not a hard day's work...a diet is a *cop out*! By seeking a "quick fix," and accepting less for myself than living up to my own standards, I alienated myself from my true values and created an inner emptiness. Dieting never allowed me to feel respect for myself...and binge eating was a statement of that self-contempt. When I began to pay my dues every single day by making the tough choices I had to make to get THIN, I developed the personal integrity I had been missing.

My bingeing had nothing to do with physical hunger. Actually, I was hungry for something other than food— MYSELF—and when that is the case, there is an empty feeling inside that no amount of food can fill up. I gave up bingeing because I replaced it with a better way to satisfy myself. I filled myself up with self-esteem, and, finally, stopped the hunger.

I never want to have another binge because I feel contempt for myself. I work very hard to avoid being the victim of the promise that a diet will work for me. I DID THE WORK...I earned my self-respect.

IV. I'M ENTITLED TO CARE ABOUT ME

I consider myself a caring, loving person. For example, if my parents needed me, I was there to help them put on a Band-Aid, even before they had time to unwrap it...or say "ouch." Like most mothers, I made *supreme sacrifices* for the welfare of my children. Even if I was dressed and ready to go to the luncheon of the year—if one of my kids sneezed— I didn't go. I wanted to be there to give them the care they deserved...*and, I never intend to let them forget that either.* When Howie needed me to work in his office, I never considered turning him down just because I **hated** working there. When someone needed me, they got me. *But what about when I needed me? Somehow, it seemed selfish to put my own name in the hat and draw it out...*

My love of family—especially at holiday time—often put me in a position to show total disregard for myself. Holidays were always lovelier, and much more enjoyable, when all of our kin were together. So every year, I invited everyone, although, it involved days of cooking, cleaning, and setting up.

My cousin, Edith, graciously accepted my invitation each year, but that was ALL she ever accepted. She wanted none of the responsibility and never volunteered to help in any way. *Perish the thought, she'd offer to cook her "specialty."* Furthermore, she'd always walk in at the last possible minute to make sure there were no chores still left undone.

Edith did, however, always bring a cake from her favorite bakery. *She had a way of carrying that cake, by the string on the box, that made me want to punch her in the face.* So to be spiteful, I never served her cake. Besides, there was always an abundance of delicious homemade goodies, so no one in their right mind would want her "bakery bought" anyway.

Immediately after dinner, as if it was her reward for not helping to set up, she departed without helping to clean up. Year after year, she showed me total lack of consideration, but I never spoke up. *After all, I felt my sole purpose on this planet was to please others.* Year after year, I simply went into the kitchen and when the clean up was finished...so was her cake. I ATE IT! *Now, I realize I was actually punishing the innocent one. Edith got off "scot free." I ate the cake...I had the guilt...I had the shame. I also had the FAT thighs... and I had done all the work!*

A few years back, I spoke up and asked for what I was entitled to. "Edith dear, I want you to be fair. I need help. I'd like you to do your share. I am not your servant." *You know what? I haven't seen her since. She isn't spending the holidays with us these days. Guess what? I don't miss her!*

I gained many a pound because I didn't consider myself

worthy. How could I possibly trouble a waitress just because she forgot to bring my salad dressing on the side? I didn't want to bother her to take that long, long walk back to the kitchen...just for me. *Of course, while I was eating too much dressing, I bet she made fifty trips back and forth to the kitchen anyway.*

Needless to say, I wouldn't even consider hurting the feelings of a waiter after he had lugged a magnificent silver tray of desserts to my table. Poor guy, I bet that tray must have weighed a ton! Patiently, he'd display each delectable selection from the fabulous array of pastries on his tray. *Like I needed an explanation to recognize an eclair?* Then in his charming European accent, he'd politely ask, "Would madame care for dessert?" How could I possibly turn him down? *What if he was on commission?*

No way I could offend him! So, if I didn't accept the dessert, I made sure, at least, he knew why. I told him the story of my life, "I was born FAT—dieted all my life—got temporarily THIN for my wedding—and started gaining weight with my first baby. Now, I'm losing weight successfully, but don't want your dessert to blow it for me." *Poor guy, all he wanted to know was whether or not I wanted dessert...and, all this time, he was still gripping that heavy silver tray.* A simple, "No thanks, couldn't eat another bite" would have done us both a big favor.

For sure, everyone has encountered a hostess who insists, "You really must try IT! I spent the whole day making IT just for you." If I don't want to eat IT...I don't. However at that point, I feel it would be quite inconsiderate not to, at least, taste IT. *After all, even I don't cook for myself any-more...but she did!.*

She's looking for the assurance I've never tasted anything better, in my entire life, then her cooking...or am ever apt to.

I give her the compliment she's seeking. I taste her "*whatever*" and rave! She goes away happy...and I go home THIN.

Caring for my friends no longer includes allowing them to force food on me. If they threaten me, "I won't eat unless you do"...believe me, they won't have anything to eat. If they try to push food on me...I push back. Doing what I don't want to do—or giving what I don't want to give—in an attempt to feel more loved—actually made me feel less worthy. So, now I don't eat—what I don't want—just to please someone else. It's not because I don't care about them. It's because I care about me!

It's not selfish to be your own person. Saying "no" to someone else merely means saying "yes" to yourself. It's not selfish to meet your own needs and ask for what you want. It's not selfish to act on your own behalf and set appropriate limits to your relationships. To be caring...it is not necessary to be the world's doormat!

All the people in my life—who were ever important to me —are still very important to me. I haven't subtracted one name from the list of those I care so much about. I've simply added one—**MINE!**

V. I'M ENTITLED TO MAKE MY OWN JUDGMENTS

My analytical mind has always been one of my strong suits. I am logical, sensible...and curious. So it seems strange that I never questioned why THIN people didn't need anyone to tell them WHAT to eat or WHEN to eat it. It's hard to believe that I didn't comprehend that THIN people didn't beat themselves up for occasionally overeating—or think that eating "forbidden" foods was the crime of the century. It's difficult to fathom that I never wondered why THIN people didn't need a diet to control their food—and I did...

I never questioned the diet system that forced me to divide my food into exactly three installments a day—and keep track of the amount of each food group I ate daily—even though, I was fairly certain that THIN people didn't have to do that. I never demanded an explanation for why they didn't attend a THIN support group meeting the night before a holiday to get instructions on how to avoid eating homemade delicacies. In fact, how come they NEVER had to go to a group meeting to get support to stay THIN?

It never occurred to me to inquire why THIN people didn't stockpile food to binge eat at night. *At diet class when I claimed, "I'm okay all day, but I need my food at night"...my instructor told me, "Save it! Save your fruit, save your milk, save your bread, and binge your brains out."* Why didn't anyone ever ask me why I needed a binge at night when THIN people didn't?

I never observed THIN folks choking down the foods they hate in an effort to lose weight. If they didn't like something, they didn't eat it. Not only that, they didn't have to follow a special program—like it or not—like I did.

I hate fruit, but at diet class, I heard, "You can't skip your fruit. Remember *undereating* is as bad as *overeating*. So, if need be, hold your nose and quickly gulp down some orange juice to fulfill your fruit requirement for the day...or else you'll be cheating." *Gosh, how could I have been so stupid? I should have known it wasn't fruit...or any other food...that would decide whether I would be FAT or THIN.*

Now, I have faith in my own judgement, so I will never again have to eat <u>anything</u> I don't like. I trust myself to SPEND my calories...not manipulate...or save them. It's just as important to be satisfied—as it is to be full. *After all, one hundred apples never took the place of one Oreo...and NEVER will!*

77

I'm through letting anyone tell me what I should do—what I should like—or what I should eat. I will never again **SHOULD** on myself—or let anyone else **SHOULD** on me— or MINE!

During the first four years of her marriage, my Barbara desperately wanted to have a baby and, believe me, I wanted her to have one. *My luck, it was financially unfeasible for her to start a family as her husband, Mark, was in medical school, and she was the sole support of the family.*

When eventually a "blessed event" was expected, she was elated! I watched—in wonder—as she enjoyed every minute of her pregnancy, and not only that, she even laughed her way all through "labor day."

Janet and I got the assignment of keeping her company until it was time to go to the hospital. For a while when the labor pains stopped...in an effort to make the baby more inclined to be born THAT day...we even sang choruses of "Happy Birthday" to Barbara's stomach. It worked!

All along, it was easy to see that Barbs really wanted a girl, even though, she insisted that her only concern was a healthy baby. She got lucky! She got both...a healthy baby girl! When the time came to take her baby home from the hospital, she beamed with pride.

For the next few weeks, she was so blissfully happy...she glowed! Nothing was too tough for her as she thoroughly enjoyed every second of motherhood.

I helped out with the "chores" for the first few weeks. Then, regrettably, I had to go back to work. *My son-in-law demanded, "Mom, you have to go back to work NOW!"* Reluctantly I left, but my little granddaughter was like a magnet...drawing me to her.

One afternoon as I was walking up the stairs to visit, I heard the baby *screaming.* Immediately, I became hysterical!

I couldn't imagine why Brenda was wailing when she was normally such a good baby. I rushed through the front door ...and my heart stopped!

Poor Barbara looked like she had been hit by a truck. Quickly, I started grilling her, "What's wrong? Has something happened to the baby? Shall I call an ambulance?" *(I pride myself on never overreacting.)* She flew into my arms, put her head down on my shoulder, and began to cry, "Mom, I don't know what I'm going to do. I'm such a terrible mother. Everyone agrees my baby is not doing what she SHOULD be doing." *What SHOULD she be doing? She's only four weeks old. Is she suppose to have a paper route...or what?*

Barbara continued, "My best friend thinks she SHOULD be sleeping more than three hours at a time and, no way, SHOULD she be getting up so often at night." The doctor said, "I SHOULD let her cry." Tearfully she admitted, "So, I'm letting her cry and I hate it." I looked at the tears rolling down the cheeks of my precious daughter. It broke my heart to see how the word SHOULD had robbed her of the **power** and the **pleasure** of caring for her own child. SHOULD had turned her *greatest joy*...into a *burden.* She had been doing fine until the world started SHOULDING on her.

My advice came fast and easy, "Trust your own judgment, Barbs, and trust the baby's judgment as well. She'll let you know what she needs. She's not the baby in the book, she's our little Brenda." She rushed into the nursery—picked up her baby—hugged her—and lovingly promised, "You don't have to be like any other baby...or do what you SHOULD do. You just have to be like YOU." These days, Brenda is doing <u>everything</u> she SHOULD be doing. She's just doing it HER WAY!

79

Me too! No longer will I allow the judgments of the DIET WORLD to dictate what I SHOULD eat...or when I SHOULD eat it.

VI.   I'M ENTITLED TO BE HEALTHY

I never addressed the issue of the connection between my weight and my health. Admitting to myself that dieting wasn't healthy would have forced me to "clean up my act." Since that little piece of "*reality*" didn't suit me very well—I chose to ignore it—hoping it would go away...

Somewhere in the back of my brain, I guess I sensed that food's prime function was to provide energy and nourishment to the body. But, that was pretty heavy stuff! It meant I would have to give up the illusion of a "quick fix" and take responsibility for my own well being. No way! It was easier to just concentrate on what my current diet did—or did not —permit. I rationalized, "I'll get THIN first, then I'll worry about my health." So, if something was on my current diet —healthy or not—I ate it.

Under the circumstances, I guess it's no surprise that I didn't win any award for grocery shopping. However, when I was buying   clothes, I prided myself on being a very educated consumer.   I read the label on every piece of clothing I even considered purchasing for me or my family. If the fabrics were not up to snuff, I simply didn't buy them. Makes it's hard to believe that, at the same time, I walked up and down the aisles of a supermarket just tossing stuff into my basket.   Brilliant!   What my family and I were wearing was far more important to me than what we were eating.

If someone I knew lost weight, I pleaded with them to tell me HOW. Of course, I never bothered to ask, "Is your diet designed to nourish my body? Are the ingredients in the foods safe? Do they contain the nutrients I need?" *I didn't care if I had to eat two prunes, a pickle and half a banana every fifteen minutes. So what? I refused to acknowledge that any danger existed. Stupidly, I was willing to sell out my own body to effect a **quick** weight loss. I didn't want to be health conscious..I only wanted to be THIN.*

When frozen dinners hit the market with only 350 calories per serving, I didn't worry about the fact that they were loaded with sodium and fat. *Who cared? Finally, control... with no cooking!* On an all protein...all carbohydrate...all liquid...or all anything else diet, I never asked, "Is my body being cheated out of what it needs?" That wasn't my problem. *After all, if the great minds of the DIET WORLD mandated, "This is the way to lose weight," who was I...a mere mortal...to disagree?*

Weight loss still remains Number One to many—while they relegate health to Number Two. A friend of mine can easily lose seventy or more pounds. I am constantly nagging him, "Lose weight because you're killing yourself." To shut me up, he points out, "Some FAT people live to a ripe old age. How do you know I won't be one of them?" *That's the dumbest thing I've ever heard! It's also true that everyone who gets hit by a truck doesn't get killed. However, I'm not willing to walk in front of a truck to find out if I am going to be one of the lucky ones to survive.*

Nor am I willing to ignore medical science and their confirmation that FAT is a contributing factor in the development of many of the major diseases that are facing us today. Pity, many people still are! Everywhere I go, I see more and more large-size shops springing up. Fashion shows with plus-size models—and magazines for big women —insinuate that if you dress it up—FAT becomes acceptable.

How can that be? FAT IS A KILLER!

The indisputable evidence is so overwhelming that no one can really deny it. Similarly, if you are lucky enough to escape physically...FAT will surely kill you emotionally!

It's true that my original reason for losing weight was the fear of open heart surgery. Now, I have an extra reason to want to be healthy—my granddaughter—my precious Brenda. *That child is truly extraordinary...the smartest, prettiest, sweetest baby in the world...and I'm not just saying that because she's mine. Trust me, it's true. But, just in case you don't believe me...ask Howie!*

I began buying her everything in sight the day she arrived. That made it almost impossible to come up with a suitable gift for her first Chanukah. After much deliberation, I suggested to Howie that we buy her a pair of two karat diamond earrings. "Are you nuts?" he chided, "Earrings that size are much too big for a two-month-old baby." *I swear that man took shopping lessons from Ebenezer Scrooge.* However, no matter what I said, Howie held firm to his resolve, so I finally agreed to buy her a smaller pair of earrings. But only after he promised, "We will buy her two karat earrings when she becomes a bride."

I want to be around to make sure he keeps that promise— to dance at her wedding—and to see her wear those earrings. Actually, forget the size of the earrings. It really doesn't matter. Believe me, the best gift I can give my Brenda is a healthy grandmother...*because then I'll force Howie to let me buy her...absolutely everything!*

My parents didn't know about fat, sodium, and cholesterol, but I do. You bet your life...health matters!

VII. I'M ENTITLED TO BE FREE

When Abraham Lincoln freed the slaves, he forgot me! I served two masters...FOOD and DIETS. It was NEVER me that dictated WHEN, WHAT or HOW I would eat. To find freedom, I made the choice to fight for emancipation. A few years ago, I had the opportunity to see what a wise choice that was...

Howie, Barbara, Mark, and I went to the home of freedom ...Philadelphia. Barb's best friend, Terri, had a baby boy and furnished us with a super reason to visit the "City of Brotherly Love."

I'm a total tourist. In Paris, I wanted to see the Eiffel Tower—in London, I wanted to see Buckingham Palace—and in Philly, I wanted to see the Liberty Bell.

We rented a car and on our way downtown, I was chattering about how excited I was to be going to see the Liberty Bell. "Although I'm not exactly sure why," I commented, "I feel a tremendous affinity toward this bell. Perhaps, it's because I am fighting for my own personal liberty." *My son-in-law immediately interjected, "Mom, I don't think that's it... I think it's probably because you're both cracked." (Rodney, you think you get no respect?) Immediately, my beloved Howie came to my defense, "Mark, that's not it either....the reason is clearly because Mom and the bell are both bigger on the bottom." Do me a favor from now on, Howie. Please, don't help me!*

While our guide was describing the history of this precious symbol of liberty, my mind began to wander. Suddenly, a shiver ran through me as I recalled that my grandparents had all come from the area in Europe where Hitler had annihilated the Jews. America had given them sanctuary...and me an opportunity to be born. *Thank you, America...for freedom.*

At the same time, a blanket of euphoria covered me from head to toe at the realization that I had also escaped a lifelong sentence in the FAT WORLD. Miraculously, my pain...shame...and...guilt...had ended. *Thank you, THIN WEIGH...for freedom.*

After seeing the Liberty Bell, we walked down the street to see an exhibit honoring the Declaration of Independence. Beautiful pictures depicted the story of the events leading up to the first fourth of July. At the end of the exhibit, a replica was provided and everyone was invited to sign it—if they would have signed back in 1776.

Leaving the DIET WORLD is proclaiming independence. However, it means fighting a personal revolutionary war—changing our belief system—taking responsibility for ourselves—and leaving the protection of step-by-step dieting...but it also means FREEDOM.

I quickly picked up the pen and signed—not just for me—but for every member of THE THIN WEIGH. We're all fighting for our personal liberty. We know we can't stop until we can look ANY food in the eye—knowing that we can control it—for until then...we can never be free.

VIII. I'M ENTITLED TO BE ME

Once in a while, we all love to put on a costume and a mask to pretend we are someone we are not. However, if we ALWAYS try to project a false image—because we feel it is more acceptable then being ourselves—our true identity can get lost. Living life without knowing exactly who we are —because we are trying to be what we are not—is not easy...

As Janet's twenty-first birthday approached, I was horrified to discover that she had never been to New York—the greatest city in the world—and the place of my birth. I asked myself, "What could be a better gift than a trip to the "Big Apple?" Nothing! *So, after checking to be sure that none of the major department stores would be closed for inventory, I reserved a room for us in a hotel overlooking Central Park. (Again, Howie was immersed in a "once in a lifetime audit" and couldn't leave town.)*

I also bought two tickets to the hottest show on Broadway, *Le Cage aux Folles. The only way I could get them was through the black market, so I prayed I wouldn't talk in my sleep and divulge to Howie how much those little suckers cost him.*

The first act of the show was absolutely enchanting and convinced me that our money had been wisely spent. The music was beautiful and I especially loved the opening number, *I Am What I Am.* What a beautiful song...and what a beautiful thought. I wondered, "Why can't I feel that way about me? Why can't I be proud of who and what I am?" True, I was FAT, but there are worse crimes in this world than being FAT...*ax murderers, tax evaders, vanilla lovers.*

To be proud of myself, maybe the first step was to figure out who I was. Was I me...or was I the image of the person I thought I **should** be? When the DIET WORLD told me WHAT I **should** like—and WHEN I **should** eat—and WHY I **should** eat it—I accepted it. Why didn't I just say, "Sorry, that's not who I am?"

Perhaps, it was because it wasn't just in my food life that I was different. I also had trouble marching to the "right drumbeat" in other areas of my life.

Even as a child, I couldn't get my body clock aligned to the right schedule. I often started my homework when most kids were sound asleep...*therefore, I always had trouble getting up in the morning.* Most kids liked to read stories...*I liked to write them.* I didn't want to study...*I wanted to socialize.* My sense of humor was natural to me...*so I couldn't imagine why everyone else took the world so seriously.*

My parents often suggested to me, "Perhaps, you could benefit from using your older sister as a role model. She never loses anything, does her homework on time, never skips her chores to have fun, and takes good care of her belongings." They didn't understand that I didn't care about such "mundane" tasks, but, nevertheless, the suggestion hurt my feelings. It gave me the impression that being *different* meant being *inadequate.* My mind heard, "If your sister isn't *peculiar,* then you must be!"

Very often my vivid imagination stood in the way of my good sense. I found it very difficult to have my "head in the clouds" and my "feet on the ground"...at the same time. Therefore, I was constantly in trouble.

One afternoon when I was about 8 years old, my dad took my sister and me to a toy store and bought us life-size dolls. It was a wonderful surprise, as well as quite a treat. *My dad didn't have the opportunity to splurge very often as it was before Master Card or Visa. You had to have cash to shop!*

At the time, we lived on the second floor of an apartment house and while running up the steps to show my mother the beautiful doll, I was daydreaming. In my mind, I was planning fascinating trips to enticing places and creating exciting adventures for my new friend and me to share. In addition, I was pondering exotic names for my doll—Penelope, Zenia, Chloe, Celeste—and, unfortunately, not paying much attention to getting safely up the stairs. So, I bumped into the railing and, sadly, my doll fell and smashed. *I'm sure my sister still has hers!*

I constantly lived with the stigma of being different and life certainly didn't improve when my younger sister, Kate, was born. Then choruses of, "How come you can't shimmy like your sister, Kate?" plagued me. *I wish I had said, "Damn it, because I'm me and can't shimmy like anyone else"...but I didn't!* I made excuses for my peculiarities until I accepted —I AM WHAT I AM—and that's all I can be.

Immediately following that revelation, a very strange thing happened. After careful scrutiny—to my amazement—I found that my role model's lifestyle seemed quite *peculiar* to me. My sister goes to the grocery store twice a week...*I only go when the light in the fridge is flashing "red alert."* She cooks every night...*I haven't cooked in so long, I've even forgotten where I keep my pots.* She watches TV every night...*I may be the only one in America who has never seen the Cosby show.* Guess what? We are both right. She is what she is—and—I am what I am.

I live by my own values these days and offer no excuses. For instance, I can't relate to the world's passion for expensive cars. My kids insist I'm crazy when I maintain that even if I won the lottery tomorrow...*from my mouth to God's ears* ...I wouldn't buy a $50,000 automobile. It would be silly because I cannot value <u>any</u> car that much. *$50,000 worth of silk blouses...yes, but a car...no!*

The DIET WORLD never gave any consideration to what I valued. They provided me with no opportunity to evaluate <u>my</u> problems, determine <u>my</u> options, select <u>my</u> solutions, or take responsibility for <u>my</u> choices. They made all the judgments, grouping me together with everyone else in the world who was overweight. Obviously, they were wrong. Everyone is not the same!

I was wrong, too! I would have taken bets that everyone in the world loved chocolate. I never even considered the possibility that someone might not feel the way I did about it. When I met Mitch...I was stunned! He loves *vanilla*!

At first, I didn't believe him. I just assumed he was joking —or worse yet—maybe, he was lying. However, during the many years we have been friends, he has proven—beyond a shadow of a doubt—he is truly a man of integrity. *Besides, his wife...my trustworthy friend, Evie...has me convinced that Mitch would never have made up a story that bizarre! I guess it's different strokes for different folks.*

At last, I'm excited about my life...because it is my life. I solve my problems with solutions that suit my needs. I've stopped trying to be super human—the perfect dieter—and have merely settled for being a THIN human being. Self-acceptance has eliminated any possibility that I will ever again have to apologize for myself. I'm good enough for ME...and...that's good enough!

IX. I'M ENTITLED TO BE A WINNER

It was crucial to get success on my side. Believe me, that's not an easy task for someone who has suffered one humiliating diet defeat after another. Of course, I lost weight—more than a million times—only to gain it back. I tried so many different diets that even my kids would ask, "What, again? Again, you're going on a diet?" *Luckily, I wasn't aware there was a limit to how many diets a person can try in a lifetime.* Sure, it was tough to continue to focus on victory after so many defeats, but it was worth it...

Shortly after I lost my weight, my special friend, Lenore, and I went out shopping. Our mission: buy fancy dresses to wear to a formal wedding. Since it was my first outing as a normal size, I was a bit nervous. I couldn't forget the agony of shopping for clothes as a size 22½ That memory made it very difficult to accept that I could simply walk into any shop and make a selection without worrying about size. *Lord knows, in the past, I had heard often enough, "I'm so sorry, darling, we don't carry your size." That's why I'm convinced that "One Size Fits All" has got to be the world's biggest lie!*

As Lenore and I walked through the front door of a little boutique, a sweet salesperson greeted me, "May I help you find your size? Timidly, I replied, "Yes thanks. I'm looking for a dressy dress in a size twelve." She answered, "Oh no, my dear!" Immediately, the blood froze in my veins and my heart stopped beating. Then—after what seemed like an eternity—she added, "I'm sure you can wear a size ten." *Instantly, I loved her! Certainly, there was no point arguing with such an intelligent woman...so I didn't.*

She helped me select a few dozen dresses to try on. *A couple of them I wouldn't have worn to a costume party...yet, there was no way I would hurt her feelings...after what she had just done for me.* She led me to the dressing rooms—which were mirrored on the outside—making it necessary for me to come out to see how I looked in whatever I had on.

In the dressing room next to mine, another woman was also trying on clothes. For some reason, everything I put on was of critical interest to her. Each time I came out of the dressing room, she had a comment to make. "Oh, that dress is beautiful. It's gorgeous. It's you!" *Trust me, in a couple of those frocks, I looked like I was on my way to the junior prom, but I gave my neighbor the benefit of her own opinion.*

Besides, she was only partially wrong. Some of the dresses were gorgeous. In fact, one of the outfits looked exactly like it had just come out of the closet of *Crystal Carrington*...and that's exactly how I felt in it. And talk about sheer delight ...I even tried on the *VERY* dress that *Erica Kane* had worn on an episode of *All My Children. Imagine me in the same dress as the "Queen of Daytime!" After all, who am I?* Yet, with each dress, I began to feel more and more like a *Crystal* or an *Erica,* and it felt fantastic.

Hours later I had tried on so many dresses, my head was spinning. So, I decided to bring Howie back to the shop with me so he could help me make this very important decision. *That way if I made a mistake, I could blame it on him.*

As I was putting on my own clothes—*which I was wearing for the last time before taking them directly to the Salvation Army*—the "fashion critic" from the next dressing room remarked, "I'm so glad I was out shopping today. I truly enjoyed your fashion show. You looked absolutely fabulous in everything you tried on. Your lovely figure does justice to any dress." For a moment, I just stood there...unable to speak. I couldn't believe she had actually said that to me. I felt so lucky!

Then, something I think Henry Ford said flashed through my mind, "The harder I work, the luckier I get." Truth is, luck had absolutely nothing to do with this victory. I survived a great deal of pain for that sweet moment. It wasn't "lucky" I was feeling...it was pride!

I had proven that no matter how tough it was to take control...I could be tougher. I had made winning my top priority—fighting one battle at a time—until, eventually, I got stronger and stronger...and food got weaker and weaker. I developed the ability to make mistakes...and not allow them to defeat me. I showed no concern for how FAST I won... or about how anyone else judged my victory. Crossing the finish line a THIN person was all that mattered!

A woman whose name I don't know—and will never know —made it possible for me to taste the thrill of victory. Make no mistake about this, it was the MOST delicious thing I have ever, ever tasted!

X. I'M ENTITLED TO BE ENTITLED

Life in the DIET WORLD led me to believe I was an inferior person. Advertising campaigns for quick weight loss programs insinuated that FAT people are not lovable or worthy just as they are. Their message is that only THIN people are winners in life. Marketing analysts—feeding on our desperation to end the pain and shame of being over-weight—try to make us believe that getting THIN will provide us with the **perfect** life...

By suggesting that THIN people have no problems...no pimples...no pain...they hope to make us even more willing to buy what they are selling. Madison Avenue "sets us up" by implying that how we look—how much we weigh—and how fast we lose weight—are the determining factors in whether or not we are acceptable.

Strategies aimed at making us believe that only by losing weight will we be loved and happy further promotes the assumption that only through dieting can we find content-ment. No wonder, we are FAT...they keep feeding us BALONEY!

FAT people are not inferior to THIN people, nor are they **bad**. Furthermore, there is much more to becoming a happy, healthy, confident person then losing weight. A change of attitude and lifestyle—as well as a complete overhaul of belief system is necessary—and a diet does not address these difficult issues.

Georgia, one of my favorite members is a recovering bulimic. One day, as she arrived for class, she greeted me, "I feel so BAD." "Are you ill, Georgia?" I asked. She looked puzzled, "No, not at all, what makes you think I'm ill? I just <u>feel</u> FAT. I ate everything I wasn't supposed to. I'm BAD. I'm worthless."

"Georgia, you can't <u>feel</u> FAT," I told her. "You can <u>be</u> FAT. Eating too much food does not make a person BAD ...only *overweight*." No way, I could convince her. She truly believes that THIN is another word for GOOD..and FAT is another word for BAD. If she doesn't eat...she's good. If she loses weight...she's good. If she eats "forbidden" foods... she's BAD.

Many others also cling to this philosophy. When Melanie joined my class, she was eager and anxious to get everything right, and listened attentively to every word I said. As she was leaving after her first class she promised me, "I am going to be **good**. I promise I'll try not to be **bad** even once this week." Her words rang in my ears all the way home.

Why? Why do these beautiful young women have to hate themselves? Why can't they know, we are not BAD people trying to be GOOD...we are FAT people trying to be THIN? We are not our bodies! We are not what we weigh! We are flesh and blood—heart and soul—human beings.

The following week when Melanie returned, she pleaded with me, "Please, Suzie, don't hate me. I was **bad** for four days." Fear gripped me. I knew the direction of the life of this precious young woman was in danger. It worried me that her emotional well being would be in jeopardy if she continued to judge herself by what she ATE. So, I made her go out the door—come back in again—and enthusiastically announce, "I HAD THREE TERRIFIC DAYS!" I admonished her, "Melanie, give yourself credit for your accomplishments and focus on your successes. That's the best way I know to build the self-esteem necessary to win the war over food."

Both of these lovely young women—and millions like them —must learn to accept that it is our bodies that are FAT OR THIN...and our choices that are GOOD OR BAD...not us.

As anorexia and bulimia reach epidemic proportions, a rage grows inside of me. I hate these insidious diseases and the society that breeds them. When it is suggested that—"image is everything"—we foster an attitude that attacks the innocent and destroys their self-esteem.

Society must find a way to change it's message....looking good IS NOT better than feeling good. Nothing is better than FEELING GOOD about who and what you are!

In an effort to make that very point one day, I asked the members of my class, "Does anyone own an original Van Gogh." Of course, no one claimed that they did. I continued, "However, if you did own a valuable Van Gogh, would you treat it with care?" Of course, everyone agreed, "We'd give an original Van Gogh the optimum care." "Well," I expounded, "I feel as valuable as an original Van Gogh." *Someone immediately corrected me and offered the thought, "With your thighs, Suzie, perhaps, you are more likely a valuable Ruebens."*

Thighs or no thighs, you bet I'm valuable. We all are...but valuable does not mean **perfect!** I love myself—because of my strengths—and in spite of my weaknesses. I no longer berate myself for what I cannot do—but, rather, I congratulate myself for all that I have accomplished.

I am entitled to feel special—not because of a number on a scale—but because I AM SPECIAL—a one of a kind original...ME!

PART

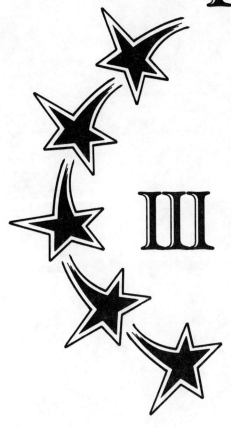

III

THE
FAT LADY
SINGS

CHAPTER
13

HEY, LOOK OUT

It's certainly no fun to have a *"fender bender"* on the highway when you've been travelling peacefully along. Yet, it happens. Maybe, we get careless and forget to look where we're going...or maybe we're just minding our own business and something smacks into us. Either way, accidents happen to everyone. Trouble is in the DIET WORLD all accidents are fatal...

Very often even the smallest indiscretion was far too major a set-back for me to overcome. I either became paralyzed with fear or guilty and ashamed of the crash. Either way, I was incapable of determining what to do next...so I quit.

Sure, it's crazy to discontinue an entire expedition because of a simple misadventure. Yet, my diet pattern was perfect or...finished!

My inability to deal with my love for "forbidden" foods was the major cause of my "head-on" collisions. In the old days when I was still food shopping for my family, I faced major problems. While unpacking the groceries, when I spied the cookies...*which I had only bought because of the children, honest...*I attempted to fight temptation and stay "legal." *Surely, even a small child knows that cookies are not on the certified list of diet foods.*

Instead in an effort to be "good," I would innocently start to nibble on the white meat turkey that I had bought to use for lunches. *Even a small child knows that although cookies are bad...white meat turkey is good.* Want to bet?

By the time, I polished off a pound of turkey—stuffing it into my face without even tasting it—I would have been much better off if I'd simply eaten and enjoyed a cookie. *Even a small child should know that a pound of turkey has far more calories then one cookie...even a big one!* But, not to worry ...I ate the whole package of cookies afterwards—because the turkey didn't satisfy me—or my craving.

In the real world, eating a cookie doesn't imply forfeiting your right to be THIN. It merely means eating a cookie. Not so for a dieter. Eating even one small cookie can produce such overwhelming guilt and shame, it leads to automatic failure.

There are no "good" or "bad" foods. I acknowledge that we must eat in portion control, but truly there is a "diet" portion of everything. *Okay, I admit sometimes it can be so small that you may need a magnifying glass to see it.* It doesn't matter. A small portion of something that is satisfying is enough!

Trying to avoid a real craving always sets up a collision. Deprivation has no place else to go except to bingeing. Well, henceforth, I refuse to be deprived of the foods I like. I refuse to be deprived of my right to self-determination. I've become an active member of the "anti-deprivation league."

Promising myself I was going to resist the foods I loved was an accident waiting to happen. No matter how firm my resolve, or how strong my determination to produce a weight loss, I found myself losing the battle to be perfect on any diet. At social occasions, when surrounded by my first one-thousand favorite foods, I vowed that I would eat only the diet stuff. Furthermore, I pledged that, at all costs, I would resist all the wonderful hor d'oeuvres...*even the little hot dogs in the blankets.* In fact, I swore I wouldn't even dare to venture into the same room as the dessert table. Of course, that was a promise I just couldn't keep.

You better believe I bent more than my "fender" out of shape, when I finally collided with the buffet table. By the time I had devoured one or two of those delectable "forbidden" goodies, my *"what the hell's the difference"* attitude took hold. After that, I stuffed myself with enough food to stock a grocery store. Miserably, I went home sick to my stomach ...and sick of myself.

Want to avoid an accident? Beware of fatigue. Trust me, it's a disaster just waiting to happen! One afternoon, I rushed into my house—exhausted—in a hurry to change my clothes—late for class—and carrying a small bag of groceries. *I had stopped at the supermarket...ugh!*

My sister, the doctor, was nagging me that I didn't get enough fiber. *Sure, finally making headway with my cholesterol and now a new worry...fiber.* Since I'm no fresh fruit lover, I bought a package of dried apricots. *There must be something in the "drying" that gives those apricots flavor. I love them!* I ripped open the bag and stuck my hand inside. Bang! No way to put the brakes on. I wound up with an empty bag.

Control must always be a positive statement made in advance. Since I had made no provision to remove the appropriate portion from the bag, I never established command. Sure fatigue was a factor. Trying to take a shortcut caused that accident!

Teaching THIN WEIGH classes, although a labor of love, claim four nights of my week—leaving me very little time for myself. Friday is my only night off so, naturally, I have become very particular about how I spend it. Since I always "dress" for class, I hate the thought of going anywhere fancy on that night. So, when one of Howard's business associates invited him to an elegant restaurant for dinner on a Friday night, I didn't feel very much like going. I had this fantasy about walking around in a pair of jeans and a shirt... with NO makeup.

Howie, for some strange reason, felt very strongly about having his wife accompany him to dinner. What choice did I have? I had to go. He didn't care that it meant I'd have to wear a dress, panty hose—and worst of all—hold my stomach in all night. *In fact, it made me livid to observe how totally indifferent he was to my plight. Go ahead, Howard, ignore my suffering. I've got a way to get even.*

Sinfully, I devised a plan to reward myself for the sacrifice I had to make on his behalf. My intention was to indulge myself by having roast duck with cherry sauce for dinner... and mousse pie for dessert. *(Bet, no THIN person can make this connection, but any "binge eater" knows exactly what I mean.)*

When we arrived at the restaurant, the maitre'd escorted us to our table. Our host then introduced us to a couple we had never met before. I am very careful when meeting new people not to tell them about my involvement with THIN WEIGH. I don't want them to feel uncomfortable about what they are going to eat, and I certainly don't want to feel obligated to always order the fish...*broiled dry.* (*Actually I live in fear that someday I will accidentally eat someone's nose. There is always one in my plate since everyone wants to see what the THIN WEIGH lady is eating.*)

Since I already knew what I was going to eat, there was no need for me to pay attention to choosing my dinner. Instead, I busied myself being charming. However, after practicing THIN behaviors for over a year, I had become somewhat of a creature of habit. Automatically, I opened my menu and glanced at it.

As I began to scan it, I noticed the specialty of the house was grouper...prepared just the way I like it. *Whoa...what a shame! If I wasn't having the duck...to be spiteful...I certainly would never have passed up that grouper. Pity!*

I didn't have much time to ponder this problem because suddenly, I felt the urge to powder my nose. Before excusing myself from the table, though, I instructed Howard to order for me. "Honey, please tell the waiter, if per chance he appears before I return, that I'll have the roast duck with extra cherry sauce, a baked potato, salad, and iced tea." Then, deliriously happy at the prospect of my upcoming feast, I gleefully went off to the ladies room. *Thanks to those damn eight glasses of water a day, I spend a lot of time powdering my nose.*

While I was gone, my sixty-seven pound weight loss must have been the topic of conversation. As I returned to the table, the gentleman I had just met addressed me, "You certainly are a beautiful advertisement for your business." I felt so wonderful...so thrilled...so proud...that when the waiter appeared a second later I heard myself say, "Please bring me the grouper." Accident avoided!

You bet your sweet bippy, everyone overeats from time to time—sometimes by accident—and sometimes on purpose. Take heart, it's not a federal offense. If you can live your whole life accident free, that's extraordinary. If you do have a mishap, however, please understand that overeating can provide a chance to learn a valuable lesson. Accidents can, if we let them, help us locate our problems, so we can seek solutions to correct them.

Of course, we must resist the temptation to berate ourselves for an insignificant misfortune. Self criticism—"You shouldn't have done it." "You never do anything right." "You can't make it."— can kill the motivation to continue and the opportunity to benefit from the experience.

What I ate yesterday doesn't matter. Each new day is a fresh opportunity to change course. Accidents don't count. Recovering—remedying the behavior that led to the collision —and being proud of handling the situation—is what produces the self-confidence that leads to success. So, just assess the damage—make the repairs—and keep on truckin'.

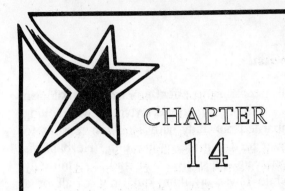

CHAPTER
14

HOW FAST WERE YOU GOING?

In this modern society of immediate gratification, where everyone has a microwave oven and eats instant mashed potatoes, I doubt *Physician's Slow Weight Loss Center* would be very popular. Everything's got to be FAST! For example, how's this for a mind boggler? I don't think that Jonas Salk received the same amount of media attention as Oprah Winfrey when he discovered a vaccine that wiped out a disease that crippled children. Oprah's feat...her announcement that she lost sixty-seven pounds—FAST. By the way, do both of these achievements sound comparable to you? They don't to me...

For some reason, we all seem to be in awe of people who lose weight FAST. Why? I view the scale simply as the equivalent of a speedometer in a car. It can't measure how well I'm driving. It only monitors how fast I'm going! *Did you know that Paul Newman is a race car driver? I bet he can drive a thousand miles an hour if he wants to. So what? That could never be what I love the most about him. No way, speed could ever compare to his magnificent blue eyes...or the rest of him...that ain't so bad either.*

Patience is a trait that we must cultivate or the constant search for instant gratification will rob us of the opportunity to develop the skills necessary to effect a permanent solution for our problem. When my friend, Myron, was selling Herbalife, he bombarded me daily with a million reasons to try it. Over and over he'd nag me by insisting, "Herbalife is the easiest, quickest weight loss I've ever had." Admittedly he was melting, while I was cranking out only a half or a quarter of a pound a week. Naturally, it tempted me, and I admit I did briefly consider trying it, except that I had made a vow to seek no more "quick fixes."

It turned out to be just as well that I held firm to my resolve. Myron eventually got tired of Herbalife...quit...and regained all his weight. Then he began a series of fad diets. Over the next year, for some reason, he never tired of trying to convince me that he was the smart one and I was the foolish one. He constantly pointed out that he was losing FAST, while I was enduring a slow weight loss.

I'd be rich now if I had a dollar for every time he urged me to try his latest diet. "This is definitely the perfect diet," he'd claim. "You are absolutely missing the boat on this one!" I wasn't buying...not this time. I just kept plugging along—minding my own business—doing my own thing—and losing weight slowly.

He never relented. He constantly badgered me with questions. "What is taking you so long? How can you possibly tolerate such a SLOW weight loss?" Then, he made the pitch. "Try my diet. Then you can lose weight FAST like me?" Believe me, it was a problem just keeping a straight face. Was he trying to tease me, or what? At that point, I had already lost fifty-six pounds, while he looked like he was making "negative" progress.

So, I decided to take the bull by the horns and boldly inquired, "Myron, how much weight did you lose last year?" He proudly responded, "About sixty or seventy pounds."

Quickly catching on to his drift, I set him up for the *"gotcha"* with a bit of flattery. "That's really outstanding, but how much did you keep off?" Timidly, he mumbled, "About five or six pounds." He's an accountant and I'm certainly no "math whiz." But, it doesn't take a genius to figure out that losing fifty-six pounds—and keeping it off—sure beats a net loss of six pounds. All of his FAST weight losses hadn't produced anything worthwhile... except for what he considers ALL important. He got to see the scale move!

With the advent of "diet club," we ushered in a whole new way of life. Now, being overweight was "organized." My friend, Hennie, and I decided to join together. Having the opportunity to get support from others who were in the same boat as we were made us very happy. Glory be, we finally had a place to go where we could be comfortable with our FAT.

Best of all, though, was their promise that all our problems would soon be over. Our membership included the guarantee that we would never be hungry again. They told us, "You can have all the string beans and mushrooms you want." *What a shame, over the next twenty years, I never ONCE got hungry for string beans or mushrooms.*

Although we both desperately wanted to succeed, Hennie was a very disciplined person...I was not. One night, as we were on our way to class, she boasted, "I've been incredibly strict all week. I followed the program EXACTLY." Talk about being dumb. Why did I pick her to go to class with anyway? Why didn't I choose someone as rotten as myself for a companion?

When we got in line to weigh-in, of course, Hennie was all smiles. I'm sure that my guilt radiated from my face. I pushed her ahead of me to allow myself more time to practice the speech I was going to give to the weigher. *No doubt, she had probably spent her whole week wondering about how I was going to do on the scale.*

Let's see, I mused, I'll her that I had out-of-town company. *Naw, I used that excuse twice before.* Maybe she would believe that I had been sick and my medicine had a lot of calories. *Nope, I'd used that one, too.* Of course, I could claim that I had been absolutely perfect. Then, indignantly allege that something was obviously wrong with her scale. *Bet, she never heard that one before.* Pity, it never occurred to me to just inform her, "This lousy diet is too tough for me. I don't want to spend the rest of my life deprived of all my favorite foods. *Besides, who in their right mind could get excited over the prospect of a lifetime of an abundance of string beans and mushrooms?*"

Abruptly, my meditation ended when Hennie stepped off the scale. She looked stricken. Horrors! She had not lost any weight. You know what that means? I was facing total disaster. I wanted to bolt and run, but there was no visible escape route. Gads, all too quickly, my turn had come. The moment for true bravery had swiftly arrived. Although I felt like I was about to face the electric chair, I stepped onto the scale. Before I even had a chance to offer up my best excuse—a miracle happened—a gift from God. I lost a quarter of a pound!

I—the **bad** one—had lost weight. Hennie—the **good** one—had not. How was that possible? How could such a thing have happened? I had no idea, nor did it really matter. We were both going home to do the exact same thing...EAT. Hennie would stuff herself because being **good** didn't work. I would gorge myself because being **bad** didn't hurt.

Pity the DIET WORLD doesn't know that losing weight is not a "good and bad" issue as much damage has been done by this concept. Anorexia and bulimia seem to have evolved in tandem with our "organized" pre-occupation with being THIN. Feeling ashamed of our inability to get THIN—coupled with the belief that diets do work—provide the atmosphere where these diseases can flourish.

Anorexia nervosa is a potentially life threatening eating disorder. Anorectics complain of feeling FAT, when in fact they can be severely underweight. In contrast to the casual dieter, they exhibit maximum willpower to give them a feeling of power and strength. Anorectics are consumed by a need for perfection and demand high performance, as well as unrealistic expectations, from themselves. They become obsessed with weight, diet, and calories. Their single goal in life often becomes to achieve control over their feelings by starving and not consuming any food. They die because they have tied their self-esteem to a number on a scale.

Bulimia is the fear of weight gain and the inability to deal with those feelings. Uncontrollable compulsive overeating is frequently followed by purging through vomiting, laxatives, diuretics, fasting, or exercise in an effort to manipulate a weight loss. These actions are frequently performed secretly and lead to feelings of guilt, shame, and worthlessness.

Bulimics suffer from a distorted image of the world and their bodies. Constantly trying to project a false image that they feel is acceptable to others—but that is uncomfortable to them—leaves them with an inner emptiness that no amount of food can fill. Their weight becomes the central focus of their lives and food becomes their method to cope with their emotional difficulties.

The DIET WORLD is the mother of these diseases. It must bear the responsibility for giving birth to them by placing the blame for obesity where it does not belong. Being FAT is not about integrity—or about character—or about self-control—but rather being overweight is about self-acceptance and shedding the unrealistic expectation that happiness can be found on a scale. I wish they knew what I know. True happiness comes from the person who lives inside of my body and not from my body's size.

I refuse to allow a scale to validate or judge me for I am not a weight....a number. I am a living, breathing human being—a paradoxical mix of strengths and weaknesses—a combination of goodness and evil...happiness and sadness... love and hate...generosity and greed...energy and idleness.

I won't let the scale confirm the quality of my choices either. *How can it? It wasn't there while I was eating.*

Put into the proper perspective, the whole issue of the scale is quite absurd. Just this morning, I lost one-hundred pounds. Want to know how I did it? The bulb for the LED read-out on my digital scale burned out. Magically, due to a fluke, did I become a <u>better</u> person...because I suddenly had a <u>smaller</u> number on a scale? Certainly not!

In my FAT life, every time I walked into my bathroom I stepped on the scale. *What did I expect to see? What could possibly have happened in fifteen or twenty minutes?* Not only that, I had this ridiculous morning routine. I'd get up and weigh myself—take a shower—and weigh myself again. *How dirty could I have been for a shower to make a difference in my weight?* And, if that wasn't enough, as a finale, I would put on my *undies* and weigh myself once more. *It was not only ludicrous, it was getting expensive. I was making a major investment in batteries for my digital scale.*

Let's suppose there was an Oscar for losing weight. Who would you give it to? Would you award it to the performer who was strict for ten perfect weeks—QUIT—and regained the weight? Or would you give the golden statue to the person who had the guts to continue...no matter what the scale said? For sure, I know who deserves it. Trust me, it's no great honor to lose weight...only to gain it back again!

In diet class, the applause was always for the BIG losers. At the end of the meeting the lecturer would inquire, "Who lost five pounds? Yea! Four pounds? Yea! Three pounds? Yea! Two pounds? Yea! One pound? Yea!" By the time they got to my quarter of a pound, everyone had either gone home or fallen asleep.

By placing the emphasis on who lost the MOST, they gave me the impression that only the BIG winners in life were worthy of attention and that being average wasn't nearly enough. Consequently, all the hard work I had done for my loss went for naught. I didn't feel like a victor. I felt like a failure!

I really don't need a scale to tell me whether I lost or gained weight or whether or not I should like myself for my choices. The power to judge me does not belong to a scale. That power is MINE.

Nobody ever has to get on a scale at the THIN WEIGH. As a matter of fact if I had my first choice, I'd pick up that "iron monster" and throw it out. Maybe, that would stop people from evaluating themselves by their weight. I feel awful when I approach a member with the greeting, "How are you?"...and the response I get is, "I lost two pounds" or "I was very bad." Damn it, I don't care about their weight. I care about them.

Of course, no one ever feels satisfied with their weight loss. No matter how much they lose in a week, it is never enough. If they lost one pound...they wish it was two. If they lost two ...then they want three. I wonder why no one ever thinks about what they didn't gain—or about how much they learned. Or how's this for an idea? Why not just accept whatever weight loss your body gives you?

The only important issue is your commitment to win the

war over food...and your firm resolve to live your THIN LIFESTYLE forever. There is one question I will NEVER answer. I will not tell anyone how much I weigh. It's not because I don't have a presentable number...I do! Rather, it's because I spent my life feeling needlessly ashamed of myself...because of what I weighed. I am not a number on a scale. I am a person—not a FAT or THIN person—a valuable person!

CHAPTER
15

I'D SWEAR WE'RE LOST

HELP! HELP! HELP! It's very scary to feel you've suddenly made a wrong turn. It's terrible not to be able to figure out where you are...or where you are going. I wish I could say that never happened to me, but in all honesty, I must confess I did get lost a few times. Perhaps, it was totally unrealistic for me to think that I would simply fight for control—WIN—and live the rest of my life happily ever after. Nevertheless, that's exactly what I thought, but I thought wrong. My control was like my life—sometimes tough—sometimes easy—sometimes a combination of both...

One Sunday morning I woke up in pain from the herniated discs in my neck. To make matters worse, I also had the world's biggest headache. I swear I felt like the top of my head was going to blow off at any moment.

All day I found myself having "food fantasies." I started talking about dinner at mid-day and, not only that, every few moments I changed my mind about what I wanted. In fact, when it was time to actually discuss dinner—*bringing in, of course, not cooking*—I couldn't get a handle on exactly what I was hungry for. I began to babble, "Let's see, I'll have fried chicken...no, Chinese food...no, pasta and pizza...no, a hot-fudge sundae." I was positively raving! I ran down the list of my first one-million favorite foods.

To avoid thinking about the pain, my brain reverted back to a time when focusing on food was my technique to block everything else out of my mind. I relapsed and gave in to my previous natural reflex of using food to avoid addressing feelings that were beyond my control. Soon, I began nibbling —lost control—and handed food a major victory. Sadly, it didn't cure the disc problem or make the headache go away. The problem was partially solved, though. I had successfully changed the subject. I didn't hate the disc or the headache, anymore. I hated myself!

Logically, I knew this was a crossroad and I had to proceed with extreme caution. If I took the wrong fork in the road ...my FAT brain would stay in charge. Surely, I didn't want to hate myself for the rest of my life. Hence, I needed to alter my approach to what I considered proper behavior. Quickly, I had to provide an environment where my THIN brain would feel comfortable and take command.

Trouble was I was having a problem trying to figure out how to instruct my brain on what was acceptable behavior... and what was not. Perhaps, I could back into it. If the opposite of acceptable is unacceptable, my job was to try to picture the most unacceptable behavior I could think of.

Understandably, it was beyond my imagination to even consider taking off all my clothes and sitting naked in the window of Neiman-Marcus. Totally inappropriate, agreed? But, how did I know that? Simple. When I was just a child, my mother made it perfectly clear that there were certain things that polite people just do not do. Accordingly, I have never even considered the bizarre notion of going shopping naked. Now, eating *out-of-control* must become as equally an outrageous behavior.

I outlined a new plan...if I lost control, I would simply take it back. In addition, I would avoid "high risk" situations until I felt in-control again. *If my aim was to avoid "slipping up" ...it would be foolish to walk around where it was slippery.* The task at hand was to persevere and recommit myself to the self-discipline required to get the job done. No problem. My desire to be a THIN person was much stronger than my desire for food.

Control is like climbing a mountain. It's beyond my imagination to ever picture myself trying to climb a mountain because of my fear of heights. Nevertheless, I have enough common sense to realize that if I was a mountain climber and fell before I reached the top, I'd have to start over at the bottom. No way I could start again from where I was when I fell. Losing control is the same.

When my FAT brain tries to control me, it screams in my ear, "You'll never make it. If it was easy to be a THIN person...then everyone would be THIN." Hearing a negative voice telling me "You can't do it" certainly makes it tough to continue. In fact, it becomes very tempting to give up. I DON'T. I use the danger signs as a warning to take extra care, not as a signal to go off course. Believe me, when I'm weak in the knees, I don't try to prove how brave I am. My goal is simply to ride out the emergency situation and survive. When it's tough, I get tougher! *I don't tempt fate by plopping myself down in an ice cream parlor...to prove how powerful I am.*

I concentrate on strengthening my sense of purpose. I recommit myself to success by using every ounce of my character to focus forward. With practice, not giving in to binge eating can become a habit, too! It takes tremendous courage to handle the hard times ...to embrace victory...when giving in to defeat would be so much easier. But, that's what

111

it takes to succeed.

At difficult times, it also helps me to remember the worst moments of my FAT life. I remind myself about how awful it felt to go to bed every night hating myself—only to wake up in the morning dreading the sight of the scale.

Once, my concern that control might slip away from me was so distressing that I actually went to the grocery store and bought two frozen diet dinners. The mere sight of them instantly reminded me of the disgust I felt when I had to eat food out of a box to control myself. It was very effective. It shocked me into immediate action. I re-dedicated myself to my THIN LIFESTYLE and began to live it to the letter of the law. *Some folks say the electric chair is not a deterrent to murder. It would be for me!*

Thank Heavens, so far, I haven't eaten those frozen dinners. I pray I never will.

Sure, getting lost can be frightening! But, not to worry. A wrong turn doesn't mean the whole trip is a flop. One day on a diet never made anyone THIN...and one day of rotten choices can't make anyone FAT.

A mountain climber may slip and fall many times before reaching the peak...but, if he picks himself up—dusts himself off—and continues...one day, he will surely be on top of the world!

CHAPTER
16

CAUTION! DETOUR AHEAD!

I thought I could write my own timetable for life, but when it didn't follow the route I mapped out for it and began pushing me around, overeating was my way to escape. Binges helped me seek relief from situations that were beyond my control...until I found more effective ways to deal with reality...

One day my sister walked into my office unexpectedly. By the look on her face, I knew that she had come to tell me something dreadful. I held my breath as she gently began to say, "I've just come from my ophthalmologist. He found a spot behind my eye." What did I know? Something was wrong with her eye, so what? That didn't sound very menacing, so I breathed a sigh of relief.

Unfortunately, my relief was premature. Sorrowfully, she went on to say, "The doctor is arranging an emergency appointment for me in the tumor department of the Bascom Palmer Eye Institute." *Tumor department? That's another story.* Obviously, I had miscalculated the danger! She could see that her words filled me with terror. Nevertheless, she delicately continued to explain that the doctor suspected the spot might be a malignant brain tumor. Hold on a minute. There MUST BE some mistake. My sister? That just can't be!

My mind raced back to all the wonderful times she and I had ever shared together...and quickly raced ahead to how much trouble I would be in if anything ever happened to her. There were so many things she knew how to do that I had never bothered to learn. I just assumed she would always be there to help me. She finished my knitting...*when I didn't know how...which was most of the time.* She has the recipes for all my favorite holiday dishes...*and I had foolishly given up cooking years before I had learned how to make any of them.* Without her, for sure, there was no way I'd ever make egg salad again. *I can never remember if it's twelve eggs for twenty people...or twenty eggs for twelve people...or something like that.* No way, I could survive if anything happened to her.

I heard this untimely news a few hours before class and I certainly wasn't looking forward to giving a lecture. I frantically searched for someone to cover for me, but no such luck. Truly, I didn't want to go to work. However, I remembered "even when it's tough—you still have to do it—if it's your job." So, off I went.

Later, I dragged myself home. Bless my kids, when they heard the news, they came over to wait for me. All of them gave Academy Award performances trying to comfort me and keep me calm. Boy, it really took a ton of courage for those kids to do that. I wasn't the only one suffering. Their hearts had to be heavy, too. It's no big secret how much they love their aunt.

After the kids left, I spent a horrendous night unable to sleep. In my whole life, I was never happier to see morning arrive. *To help you understand just how important my sister is to me, let me mention that I cancelled my regular hairdresser's appointment to accompany her to Bascom Palmer.*

I was a nervous wreck, but tried not to show it, as we

114

walked into the hospital. The patient representative greeted us in the lobby and escorted us to an examining room. *I'll always bless them for letting me stay with her instead of making me cool my heels in the waiting room.* The medics began a million tests. About midday, they recommended that we take a break for lunch. They explained that my sister needed a full stomach for the next procedure as it involved a dye injection. As she and I were walking toward the elevator to go to the cafeteria, I spied a cart loaded with goodies—exquisite brownies, magnificent cookies, gorgeous pretzels, beautiful candy...all my favorites. *Remarkable eyesight...especially since I wasn't even wearing my glasses! Wow, that stuff looked like just what I needed to get me through this nightmare. After all, junk food is the ultimate pain reliever...right?*

Quickly, I admonished myself, "You are here to take care of your sister and she needs real nourishment. Forget your nonsense. The cafeteria is a much better choice for her." Somehow, we managed to choke down something to eat and quickly returned to the examining room.

Blissfully, shortly thereafter, the technicians finished their battery of tests. Then, after what seemed like two or three centuries, the ophthalmologist finally appeared to examine her. I'm sure that while he was gazing into her eye before rendering his final diagnosis, I stopped breathing.

Unquestionably, at that moment, I truly needed a BIG favor from God and hoped I still had one coming. Silently, I began to pray, "Dear God, help me. In the past, I know I've annoyed you by repeatedly asking you to assist me on the scale. Please don't hold that against me NOW and I promise I'll never bother you again by asking for a weight loss that I didn't earn. Merciful God, I'm begging you to let my sister be okay."

115

After listening to their medical "mumbo jumbo" for an eternity—and not understanding a single word that anyone said, I couldn't stand it for another second. So, I interrupted the action and pleaded for someone to tell me what was going on. Compassionately, the doctor responded by revealing, "I'm promising your sister that everything is going to be all right. She does NOT have a malignant tumor—just the equivalent of a *freckle*—at the back of her eye. I promise that it is nothing that will ever harm her."

Joy spread through me from the top of my head to the tip of my toes. I was delirious...overjoyed...ecstatic. She was out of danger. What a delicious moment. Talk about brilliant! Gosh, I couldn't have been any smarter when I decided not to eat the junk food. Now, I was free to enjoy this glorious moment to the fullest. Victory was mine. I had beaten food this time.

Sure I had been in pain...and pain hurts...but sometimes there is no way to avoid it. Someone very precious to me had been in jeopardy, but I had survived the crisis by using my inner resources. I didn't "cop out" with junk food in an attempt to hurl myself into oblivion. By enduring the pain—without seeking a "sugar coated" escape—I earned the right to jubilation!

I didn't always choose to side-step a detour, though. There were times when I chose to wander a bit off the beaten track. For example, my Steve's college graduation. *Finally, he had his MBA...and the time had come for him to get a... JOB! For a parent, that milestone is the equivalent of getting an extra large pay raise.* I gingerly approached Howie and suggested that we make Steve a graduation party at his favorite restaurant. *Of course, Mr. Practical replied, "Are you crazy? A party like that will cost us a bundle." Truly, I'm not just another pretty face. I know how to handle my guy. I*

*calmly pointed out to him, "Not nearly as much as another
year's college tuition would cost."* He quickly agreed to give
the party.

A baseball theme was a MUST. *What else would be fitting
for the world's most avid Chicago Cubs fan?* In fact, everything had to be special, so I carefully chose a menu that
included all the foods Steve loves. However for dessert, I
ordered MY favorite—seven layer cake. *I didn't even feel a
bit guilty about that either. Why not MY favorite? After all, I
had come up with the idea for the celebration!*

The party was super. Nothing is quite as wonderful as
being surrounded by all your "nearest and dearest" friends
and family. Even my cousin, Martin, flew in from Dallas to
surprise Steve. Although, I was truly enjoying every aspect
of the evening, no matter what else was happening, I
couldn't get the cake out of my mind.

When the big moment finally arrived to serve dessert, my
face lit up at the glorious sight of that magnificent cake!
*Thank Goodness, not even a whole year of living like a THIN
person had diminished my love for food.*

The waiters started cutting *generous* pieces of cake. *Sure,
what did they care if I had leftovers to take home?* I waited
—not very patiently—until finally they put one slice of cake in
front of me and one slice in front of Martin. I ate mine—
savoring every mouthful—then noticed Marty had not even
touched his cake. As incredible as it sounds, he claimed that
he didn't want any dessert.

Beats me how anyone can pass up seven layer cake—and I'll
never know exactly why he did—because I didn't ask! I just
slid his slice of cake in front of me so fast that heads spun
around. From all areas of the room people roared, "Are you
insane? You can't eat another piece of cake!" Someone
even tried to remove the second serving from in front of me,

117

but to no avail. I insisted, "You bet your sweet bippy, I'm going to eat it. This is a day that I've dreamed about for a long time. My baby has graduated from college. Our financial nightmare has ended. And, I'm going to rejoice... MY WAY!" I ate the two pieces of cake and enjoyed every morsel.

I've often asked myself what I would have done if I'd been on a diet that night. After all, by eating cake, I'd hardly been one-hundred percent perfect. No doubt, two pieces of cake would qualify for "blowing" any diet. To be absolutely honest, given my past history, I'm sure I would have continued to binge my brains out until the next fad diet arrived.

A THIN LIFESTYLE is different. The morning after the party, I returned to my "norm." I ate one slice of light toast for breakfast...a sandwich on light bread for lunch...a quarter of a chicken and baked potato for dinner—my typical Monday routine.

If I could live that night over and make that choice again, would I act the same way? ABSOLUTELY! It's the direction that I'm traveling - not what I do along the road - that is important. My goal in life is not to avoid cake forever...it's to live a THIN LIFESTYLE forever.

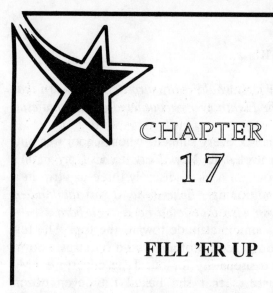

CHAPTER
17

FILL 'ER UP

Ever since I can remember food was my grand passion...an escape from pain...comfort in times of crisis...a companion when I was lonely...a hero to rescue me from misery. How foolish! FOOD IS FOOD...that's all it is. Unquestionably, the basis of my compulsive eating was my relationship with food—and not the foods I was eating. So, no matter how badly I wanted to lose weight, I could not stop overeating until I examined the needs food was satisfying for me. Then, I found better ways to gratify my emotional hungers...

FOOD IS NOT LOVE

Walking into my mother's kitchen was like having a giant bear hug envelop me from head to toe. The way her face would light up when she saw me come into the room made me feel like the most loved and treasured person on the face of the earth. I can still picture her standing there preparing all of my favorite dishes. As long as I live, I know that cherished memory will remain in my heart.

Holiday or birthday time she'd really move into high gear and cook non-stop to prepare a feast that she felt was worthy of her family. *It would really surprise me to learn that even King Henry the Eighth ever encountered a more majestic feast.*

During my childhood, every summer when school was out, my family and I traveled to New York to visit my mom's relatives. We set out on a nice, leisurely three day trip in a car without air-conditioning. *Believe me, it was the kind of outing that made you wish that you'd never been born.*

My mother had a simple attitude toward the trip. She felt that if we had enough food, nothing could harm us. So in January, she started preparing for our June departure. My conservative estimate is that she baked fifty-seven dozen cookies...fixed nine roast chickens...forty-three sandwiches... thirty-two hard boiled eggs...*and a partridge in pear tree.* Her rationale was, if per chance, we got stranded between Florida and New York, for any reason, at least, we wouldn't starve. *Forget Stuckey's or Howard Johnson's. She loved us far too much to trust our stomachs to strangers.*

On the morning we left, when my Dad turned the key in the ignition, we began eating. Before we crossed the state line, ALL the food my mom had prepared for the entire trip was gone. *That has to be the explanation for why, to this day, whenever we go on a car trip, the minute Howie turns the key in the ignition—I'm hungry!*

My mom's attitude toward food never changed. When I was forty, my gynecologist discovered my uterus and ovaries had "spoiled" and I needed a hysterectomy.

Trust me, at no time was my life ever in danger. Nevertheless, my poor mother worried non-stop and complained constantly that my doctor obviously had no compassion for the sick. She didn't understand why after the surgery, the doctor didn't permit me to eat or drink anything for two days. No way, I could persuade her the reason it was done was to prevent gasses from forming in my stomach. She was thoroughly convinced that it was actually an attempt to spite her.

All day, she stood at the foot of my bed wringing her hands and worrying that I wasn't eating. *Truly, love is blind. She never noticed that I was more than seventy-five pounds overweight and, surely, no reason existed for her concern that I might starve to death in just two days.*

When the doctor finally gave the "food okay," my mom inquired, "Mamala, what can I bring you?" *She ignored the fact that I was on the American plan at the hospital and, of course, all my meals were part of the package deal. .* In truth, I felt so wretched that the last thing on my mind was what I wanted to eat. But, I loved her so much, there was no way I could refuse to let her feed me. So to humor her, I requested that she bring me raisin toast and hot chocolate. She smiled remembering that was exactly what she had always given me as a child when I was sick.

I, honestly, didn't expect her to bring it as she lived miles and miles away from the hospital. Would you believe that sainted woman made the toast—wrapped it in aluminum foil —put it in a towel—then stuffed it into an insulated bag—and accompanied by a thermos of hot chocolate—carried it to the hospital? Why? Simple. She LOVED me.

And, I learned from her example. At age twenty-four, my Janet had to have her tonsils out. *Can you believe that? Almost the president of IBM and stricken with something as infantile as bad tonsils.* Naturally, I didn't want her to be alone when she went down to surgery. So, in a moment of weakness, I volunteered to come to the hospital to be with her before the procedure, although getting up at 5:00 AM is hardly my first choice. *I bet the first specialty they teach in medical school is "early rising." It must be...because all these damn procedures begin at dawn.*

No way, though, did I want to face food at that hour. So, I hurried off to the hospital without breakfast. I was a walking zombie in the visitor's room...half asleep...awaiting word that she was okay. I admit it wasn't all that traumatic. Her doctor was a friend of ours and I felt confident that she was in very good hands. I sipped a cup of coffee—fantasized that everything was all over—and wished I could go home and take a nap.

As soon as the doctor arrived to tell me that Janet had come through her ordeal with flying colors, I was suddenly anxious to see my daughter. Knowing how squeamish I am, he advised me to wait a bit before going up to her room. He cautioned me that she still had her IV connected. No way, no waiting, I was impatient to see my baby and ignored the doctor's advice. *Howie's only comment, "So what else is new?"*

As I reached the door of Janet's room, the orderlies were just bringing her up from the recovery room. She was lying on a gurney, looking very pale, very frail, and very unhappy. My poor child!

Instantly, I was hungry. No ravenous! These medical matters are not my bag and I don't handle them very well. I thought, "What I really need is a something to eat to help me ignore what happened to Janet." I admit it was cowardly, but so what? Then, I took another look at my little girl lying there so bravely. What kind of example would I be setting for her? She was handling her ordeal—without food—and if she could do it—why couldn't I?

When it was time for her to be discharged, I offered to take her home from the hospital and care for her. *I'm sure this time, they will have no choice. That damned "Mother of the Year" award will have to be bestowed upon me.* When we arrived at Janet's place, she went right to bed, of course. Gosh, I hated the way she looked...so pale, so uncomfortable, so unhappy...and so THIN. Therefore, every few minutes I went into her room and asked, "Mamala, what can I do for you? Do you want soup? Do you want ice cream? Do you want Jello? Do you want cereal?" *So what if she was sleeping? I had to take care of her!*

It hurt her too much to talk, so she finally wrote me a note. "Mom, do you want to leave me alone?" Obviously, I was annoying her. Know why? Simple. I LOVED her.

Amazing, my mother passed it down to me...and I went ahead and passed it right along to my kids. A few years ago, I had a vicious flu, which made me feel so wretched that I actually prayed for death. My children all generously volunteered to take care of me, but there was a flaw in their magnanimous offer. They all had to go to work. So, instead of actually being with me, they made a pact to take turns calling to check up on me.

First up...Barbara. "Mom, before I begin my day, do you want me to bring you anything for breakfast?" I appreciated her concern, but answered, "No thanks sweetheart. Don't worry, I'm okay." Next call was from Janet. "Do you have anything to eat for lunch? I'm sure I can take a few moments off and run over with some chicken soup if you don't." *How? I don't know. Her office is about twenty-five miles from where I live.* "No thank you precious, I'm doing just fine." Last came Steve. "What's up for dinner, Mom? Need anything? On my way home from the office, I can stop and get you something. Want Chinese, Italian, KFC?"

"Honey, thanks for the offer, but Dad is taking care of those arrangements."

Of course, I appreciated their interest. Why wouldn't I?

123

It feels terrific to know that your family really cares about you. Sure, I was grateful for their attention, but I was also amused. Know why? At no time did anyone ever ask me if I needed an aspirin...a tissue...cough syrup...or a throat lozenge. Guess what? They are my kids and they LOVE me!

Truth is that my mom, my kids, and I are all wrong. **LOVE IS LOVE...AND FOOD IS JUST FOOD.**

FOOD IS NOT ANESTHESIA

After I lost my parents, it was not my habit to visit their graves at the cemetery. *My mother was such a fun person, I have no doubt that she refused to stay there...or let my Dad remain there either. I'm confident that she has located a party somewhere and both of them are having a terrific time.* However, one day something special happened that made me want to pay tribute to them...

My beautiful granddaughter is named for my parents... Beatrice and Harvey. In honor of that special occasion—her naming party—I filled my house with flowers...roses and heather. Roses—my mother's favorite flowers—were an obvious choice. In fact, she loved them so much that she always wore the essence of roses as perfume. Forever, whenever I smell that fragrance, it will remind me of her. Heather was another logical choice. That's the baby's middle name—given in honor of my father. *Howie was afraid that they would have to fly the heather in from the moors of Scotland. He got lucky. My local florist had some in stock.*

The morning after the party, as I looked at the beautiful baskets of flowers, I felt an overwhelming desire to bring them to the cemetery. It seemed like just the right way to acknowledge that life continues. After all, now, beautiful Brenda Heather had arrived to replace my loss.

It was a tough moment as I kneeled to place the flowers on their graves. Why were they there when I wanted them to be with me to share the excitement of the newest addition to our family? Why had the chance to see the wonder of what they had started been denied to them? It wasn't hard to imagine how they'd both burst with pride if they could see Barbara...all grown up...and a mother!

Why did I lose them so young, anyway? It wasn't fair. We should have had more time together. I was angry because it was so unfair.

As I stood up, a sharp hunger pang almost knocked me off my feet. I recognized it immediately. It was emotional hunger...and it came as no surprise. For years, food had functioned as my way to stifle my feelings. At that moment, I wanted my grief to go away and, in times of trouble, a binge had always been my "escape route." Maybe, now, it could help me obliterate the pain—or, at the very least—help me to deny it.

The thought was tempting until I remembered that bingeing had brought me more suffering than any of the real pain I had ever tried to suppress.

No bingeing was necessary this time. Luckily, I had learned a valuable lesson about pain. There is absolutely no way to eradicate it...and no need to deny it. Besides, it is unrealistic to expect life to be pain free.

True, I had lost something very precious—and that hurt me very much—but that had nothing to do with food. What could food do for me, anyway? At best, it could soothe me, numb me, or distract me. Forget it! I certainly didn't want any of that.

So, right here and right now, I had to face my feelings. I

will always miss my mother and dad. However, blocking out that grief with a binge would limit the extent of my happiness. I reminded myself, "The same wall that keeps out pain ...keeps out joy." No way did I want that. After all, I was going home to the delight of my first grandchild.

Sorry food, I don't need you anymore. I can handle my grief myself. **FEELINGS ARE FEELINGS...AND FOOD IS FOOD.**

FOOD IS NOT COMFORT

Sometimes life can be very grim and there is nothing deadlier to determination then negative feelings. The herniated discs in my neck cause me a lot of suffering. *Unfortunately for those around me, I never suffer in silence. When I am miserable...the whole world is miserable.* Although, my physical condition has curtailed many of my activities, I try not to let it stop me from doing what I especially love to do...

One Friday, my friend, Elaine, and I decided to make a day of it and go shopping. It was exciting because I love *shopping* almost as much as I love *chocolate!* Our plan was to browse in the charming boutiques and art galleries in Coconut Grove. *While in the neighborhood, of course, if necessary, we'd force ourselves to cover the nearby major malls.*

We spent a wonderful day, except that I came home absolutely exhausted, and in a considerable amount of pain. My neck hurt so much, I cancelled our dinner plans. Instead, I stayed home with Howard...and my heating pad.

The next morning, I fully expected to feel better, but I didn't. I developed a bad case of "*poor me*"...and plunged into a blue funk.

Sunday, our plan was to go to an art show with our friends,

Norma and Bobby. I wasn't feeling any better, but I certainly didn't want to be a wet blanket. Thus, I made the ultimate sacrifice and decided to go. When we got there, immediately, I noticed the magnificent works of art—*brownies, muffins, pizza, french fries, corn dogs.* Norma tried to point me in the right direction by making me aware of the fact that the show also had paintings, sculptures, and crafts. However, in my current frame of mind, I couldn't have cared less.

After years of using a "food fix" as an escape valve from distress, I was chafing at the bit to eat everything in sight. My discomfort became the "trigger" that sent me seeking a food bandage for my "*boo-boo.*" For years, I had always found solace in food. So, why not now?

Hold on a minute. Was it necessary to limit myself to the old behaviors of the past? Just because that's the way I used to act, does that make it appropriate? Even though triggers remain strong for years, is that a reason to give in to the food cues? Am I bound to the past, forever? Nope!

I analyzed the situation. Enduring my giant case of "*I don't feel well*" was tough. I told myself, "Sure, under the circumstances, indulging in food seems fully justified. After all, you've been suffering all weekend." Then, I asked myself, "Yet, does this torment even come close to comparing with the humiliation and disgust of being FAT?" I quickly answered myself, "It's not even close. Those days of my life were more painful than ANY physical condition I've ever had to endure."

So, I corrected my original thought, "You deserve better than a binge. Okay, you have pain, but so what? A binge can't help make you feel better. In fact, you'll have *twice* the pain, not *half* the pain. You'll still have your physical suffering and you'll be adding the guilt and shame of the binge."

I controlled my eating. I didn't give in to the *"poor me"* syndrome. I found the courage to ignore the trigger by simply refusing to respond to it. I concentrated on victory. I took another look around at the available food. Know what? I didn't see anything that I wanted more than I wanted to be THIN. Food is not a pain killer. **COMFORT IS COMFORT...AND FOOD IS FOOD.**

FOOD IS NOT A CELEBRATION

The day after Barbara and Mark's wedding, I began my campaign to persuade them to have a baby. I ignored the obvious. He was in medical school and couldn't support a baby. Therefore, she had to work and couldn't care for a baby. *But, that was their problem. Why should I suffer?* Every day for four years, I emphatically told her, "I want you to have a baby." *When I couldn't reach her in person, I left an anonymous message on her answering machine.* Believe it or not, after four years of getting ready, when the moment actually arrived, it surprised me...

One afternoon, Barbara called my office and invited Howie and me to go out for dinner. Her timing couldn't have been worse. The following night, I was having company for dinner and had a million chores to do...including the awful grocery store. To make matters worse, I wasn't feeling very well, so I asked for a rain check.

I left work a bit early to rest up. While sitting around waiting for Howie to get home, Barbara called again. "Come on Mom, let's all go out together," she said. "Mark and I will even go to the grocery store with you after dinner." *I should have known something was up. What normal person volunteers to go to the grocery store?"* She sounded so anxious to see us, of course, I couldn't turn her down.

When we arrived to pick them up, Barbs and Mark came rushing down the steps. As I got out of the car to greet them, she took my hand and put the positive pregnancy test in it. WOW! Talk about excited. Talk about delighted. Talk about happy. I was all three.

Instantly, I wanted cake and ice cream! Know why? I've always liked to share my good news with my three dearest friends—*Ben, Jerry and Sara Lee.* Want to hear something amazing? This time, the announcement was so scrumptious that even an entire Ben and Jerry's franchise could not have made that news any happier.

For the next nine months, we anticipated the biggest celebration in our family's history. One thing for sure, there was no way I was going to take a chance that I'd wreck this "happening" with the burden of having to lose weight. I vividly recalled how FAT had ruined the days which led up to Barbara and Mark's wedding. *Don't even think about it this time, FAT. I'm writing a new script for myself.*

There is no way I'm going to be spending my time promising myself every day that I will stay on a diet. No way, I'm going to bed every night hating myself for breaking that promise. *Besides, I won't have time for any of that. I'll be too busy shopping for the baby!*

When the big day arrived, we took Barbara to the hospital early in the afternoon. I figured she'd have the baby in a few hours and then we'd all go out to dinner. Well, Barbs didn't exactly follow that plan. We were still sitting around the waiting room at 8:00 PM...and stomachs started growling. *Believe it or not, there were eighteen people in the hospital awaiting the arrival of our "blessed event."*

129

I listened in amazement as the dinner discussion began. Obviously, no one wanted to miss the magic moment, so "take out" was in order. But what? Everyone had a different opinion, "I want subs—I want Chinese food—I want ribs—I want a catered meal with champagne and caviar." *Can you believe to some people even the birth of a baby is not more important than food?*

Howie turned to me and asked, "What do you want, honey?" Trust me, I'll never answer an easier question. "I want a healthy baby. I want my Barbara to be okay. I want a celebration! Know what else, Howie? I don't particularly care what I eat."

Shortly, thereafter, the magic moment finally arrived. Lucky me, I got exactly what I'd ordered—my beautiful Barbara was beaming! Why not? She was the proud mother of a gorgeous, healthy, baby girl!

No matter how long I live, for the rest of my life, I will remember that moment. But, honestly, I can't recall what I had for dinner that night!

Cake and ice cream are delicious...but not as delicious as a real celebration. **JOY IS JOY...AND FOOD IS FOOD.**

FOOD IS NOT ENTERTAINMENT

Even in her heyday, I doubt that Bette Davis got the kind of attention I used to give to food. I treated selecting my next meal as if was the most important event of the century. The discussion about Saturday night dinner began on Monday morning and was the topic of conversation all week long. *I swear Howie and I bought our wonderful new townhouse with less deliberation than I used to give to selecting a restaurant.* I wasn't the only one...

Very often after class, several of my members join me for dinner. Since I eat out so often, I usually leave the choice of where we're going up to them. Well, you'd think that selection was the most important decision ever made. "Let's have Chinese food." "No, I don't want Chinese, I had it five days ago." *Imagine remembering it was five days ago. I can't remember what I ate yesterday.* "Well, how about Bar-B-Q?" "Naw, I don't feel like Bar-B-Q. Whenever we go there, I want the ribs and that's not the right choice for me." This literally could go on for hours if I didn't remind them, "Hey, I'm hungry and tired. Pick a place already and let's go."

Boredom ever make you eat? It did me! If I was alone, nothing could be more entertaining than a "chocolate covered evening." A crummy T.V night? Could you ask for a more pleasant way to pass the time than raiding the fridge? Give me a break, am I not entitled to a little enjoyment out of life? Sure!

But, honestly, how long does that happy, full feeling last? It's fleeting at best. The bitter taste of self-hatred and despair quickly replaces the fabulous taste of the food. Those exciting bites of food, always bit me back with guilt and self-disgust.

Sure eating is fun, but pleasure is not happiness. Quite the contrary. Although food brought me some delicious moments, it robbed me of the opportunity for real enjoyment. By restricting myself to the small world of the refrigerator, I stayed bored and turned to food for relief. It became a vicious cycle. I never saw that the true problem was boredom—not hunger.

There's a whole big world out there. Yet, the FAT mission in life is like the "prime directive" of *STAR TREK*—seek out and explore all new restaurants. It used to be my life's work to make sure that I ate in every new bistro in town, while ignoring everything else that life had to offer!

Recently, I took an informal survey of my friends, family, and members. I asked, "Have you ever seen the beautiful new library and museum in downtown Miami? Have you gone to the theatre, art shows, ballet, opera—or you name it —recently?" Nope! But, they knew the exact location of every new restaurant in town. And, that's not just unique to Miami. My aunt and uncle lived in New York all their lives. Yet, neither one of them have ever seen the Statue of Liberty. However, you can ask them about all the finest eateries in town...and they'll have the answers.

Food doesn't deserve all that acclaim. Food is not entertainment. It cannot make us laugh. It cannot tell us jokes. It cannot be dramatic. Food never won an Academy Award, an Emmy or a Tony...and it never will. **FUN IS FUN...AND FOOD IS FOOD.**

FOOD IS NOT STRESS

Recently, I saw this terrific movie on the nostalgia channel, *The Perils of Pauline.* Talk about mishaps, poor Pauline had one disaster after another. She was constantly in trouble. In the short span of one film, we find her tied to a railroad track with the train coming...hanging by her fingernails from a cliff...or inside a burning building with the flames leaping all around her. Luckily, however, she had a handsome hero who always showed up just in the nick of time to save her. No doubt about it, my handsome hero was FOOD...

It served as my bridge over troubled waters, a barrier to protect me from harm, an old reliable friend, or a stress reducer. If there was too much traffic on the expressway... a binge. If I didn't get my own way...a binge. If something happened beyond my control...a binge. If I had too much to do or not enough to do...a binge. If I was disappointed or hurt...a binge. If I had to accept something that I didn't like ...a binge.

If something couldn't be fixed...just fix it with food. If I was afraid to deal with something...it was easier, instead, to deal with food. And, of course, in times of stress, what could be more useful then the ultimate tranquilizer?

Sure, everyone has periodic times of stress and pressures in their lives. Not me! I used to spend ALL my time worrying...about everything! I had a million real or imagined problems and they all served as obstacles to my losing weight.

Having the title of "world class worrier" was no great honor. Besides, worry never solves problems. So, I taught myself a valuable tension-relieving technique. I learned to RELAX! I lightened up and stopped taking everything so darn seriously. I stopped trying to control my life and let go of my desire to manage the world. I replaced stress with fun.

Truth is, food was never a good stress manager, anyway. A realistic expectation is much better. Developing the attitude to accept life on a day to day basis really works. If something is beyond my control, I don't try to control it. If something happens that I can't change, I don't try to change it. If I have to accept something that doesn't go my way, I accept it. I don't always like it—but accepting doesn't mean liking—it merely means accepting. If I do something someone else doesn't like, so what? If it's okay with me, it's okay!

I no longer insist that life run smoothly all the time and that I am always comfortable and happy. Sure, we all have troubles, but food isn't the solution. Believe it or not, even chocolate cannot solve problems...*not even the small ones.* Quite the opposite, food prevented me from locating the

133

origin of the problem and finding ways to eliminate or cope with it.

I have proof that food can't solve problems. Over and over, I've asked this question in my classes, "What food helps you solve your problems?" I have no answer. I never will...because the only problem that food can solve is hunger.

Binge eating merely acts as a temporary stop-gap. It never addresses the problem...never provides a solution...and never allows us to be THIN.

A more effective way to deal with pressure is one problem at a time—one day at a time—trusting yourself and your ability to handle your daily life. **PROBLEMS ARE PROBLEMS... AND FOOD IS FOOD.**

FOOD IS FOOD

The DIET WORLD taught me to sneak food...save it... trade it... store it...exchange it...manipulate it—but never to be comfortable with it. They persuaded me that some foods were bad and cautioned me to avoid them. Well, they were wrong. Food is not bad. It is what we use it for that can be destructive...

Obviously, what I learned wasn't enough...because it NEVER worked. It finally became impossible to ignore the fact that my "diet mentality" was actually making me FATTER every year. By blaming my condition on certain foods and accepting that all I had to do was eat "non-fattening" foods to get THIN, I stopped looking beyond food for the true reasons I was overweight.

Originally, I decided to stop dieting in an effort to save my health. Soon, it also became more and more apparent that staying FAT was tougher than getting THIN. Finally, I began an honest "fact finding" mission to learn about food...

and about myself. My most important discovery—FOOD IS JUST FOOD.

I was very apprehensive when it was time to translate the language of dieting into freedom of choice. It terrified me to think that I might confuse permission to eat what I wanted with permission to binge eat. But, I soon discovered that eating what you want—whenever you CHOOSE it—is not the same as eating as much as you WANT—every time you WANT it.

Having the right to determine what, when, and how I was going to eat was my first step in learning self-trust and becoming a THIN person. Ironically, it was freedom of choice that gradually enabled me to overcome overeating. Pity, freedom of choice is what I had so little of in my diet life.

In a world full of "unlimited" foods—and no responsibility for self-regulation—volume was always the name of the game. In a world full of "forbidden" foods—binge eating was inevitable because there was no alternative method for selecting these foods.

In the past, I thought that happiness was permission to eat anything I wanted—anywhere—anytime—and in any quantity. Truth is, now I understand that what I really yearned for was the right to exercise my freedom of choice and for the chance to take responsibility for my own life.

Giving myself permission to eat ANY food helped me to understand that no amount of food can ever abolish deprivation. When I realized that I could choose to eat the foods I loved, the desire to eat them constantly eventually dissipated. Then, I automatically developed the ability to make the choices that would allow me to be THIN.

FAT people can't do that. For them, volume is still the name of the game because they have never found an adequate way to satisfy themselves. So, when "diet" food arrived on the scene with fewer calories than regular food, no dieter even considered being rational...and settling for less. They just ate twice as much.

After I had already left the DIET WORLD, one night, I noticed my friend, Margie, had brought her diet bread and diet salad dressing to the restaurant with her. Her dedication to purpose impressed me until I observed how she handled her meal.

While we were waiting to order, the waiter brought over a delicious looking basket of sour dough rolls. They looked so luscious that I took one out of the basket and put it on my bread plate. *(Remember, never eat anything out of it's original container.)*

Even though the roll looked tempting, I decided to wait for my salad to arrive before eating it. Margie ate one slice of her diet bread while we were waiting. When the salad arrived, Margie carefully poured her diet dressing on her salad...and ate an additional slice of diet bread.

We ordered. I chose a small lobster—with no stuffing—and a baked potato. Margie chose prime rib and a stuffed baked potato. After the salad, she finished her additional two slices of diet bread, while I opted to wait for my dinner.

I ate my lobster and potato, which was sooooo good, enjoying every last bite. She, too, finished everything, although, I swear her prime rib was so large, it was hanging over the side of the plate. Then, as a finale, she had a sour dough roll.

When it was time for dessert, we both passed. *They didn't have anything interesting in chocolate!*

Let's recap. She had four slices of diet bread—and one regular roll—*I had one roll.* She had high calorie roast beef —*I had low calorie lobster.* She had the stuffed potato—*I had a plain potato.* Tell me, what good is eating diet food if you are overeating? No good! It isn't how we save our calories that counts, it's how we spend them! My goal is not to manipulate food. My goal is to control it.

Recently, I have fallen in love with DOLE WHIP. Ever taste it? It's a whipped fruit, the consistency of yogurt—*which I hate*— but with a much better taste. I can't find it everywhere and when I do, I grab the chance to enjoy it. One evening, Howard and I were walking on the boardwalk along the beach and I spied a place selling DOLE WHIP.

One portion has eighty calories—roughly the equivalent of one and half pieces of fruit. My FAT brain got excited and immediately called to my attention, "You haven't had any fruit today. Not only that, but you didn't have any yesterday either. You know on most diet programs, you can have three fruits every day. Lucky you, now, you are dealing with six fruits." Thinking fast, my FAT brain calculated that I could have four portions. Even if I only had two, though, I'd still be two ahead of the game!

Sounded terrific until my THIN brain spoke up, "Who do you think you're kidding? You know that only ONE portion is appropriate. I've never seen you eating two lunches or two dinners." You're right, THIN brain. I'm willing to settle for one portion of a food I love...and a THIN body, too. In fact, I just can't ask for more than that!

For years, I thought food knew its ethnic origin. I suppose that was just another fabrication the DIET WORLD used to keep me in line. No Chinese, Italian, Mexican or French food allowed! I guess they felt giving me "*plain*" food would keep me out of trouble. Well, maybe, ethnic food was their problem, but it wasn't mine. The fact that it was "forbidden" was what messed me up.

Let's face it, if I wanted Chinese food, I was going to have it...whether anyone else liked it or not. Unfortunately, as long as it was cheating, I had only two choices: behave myself or "don't behave myself."

Of course, it was the "*don't*" behavior that was fattening. I'd sit down at the table and polish off a bowl of noodles before I ever saw a waiter. Then with my soup, I'd finish another bowl of noodles. No way, I could ever pass up a Pu-Pu platter...*served for two only.* So, I shared it with Howard...*who doesn't eat Chinese food!* Then, dinner, and, of course, ice cream. *Chinese ice cream tastes better and comes with a wonderful fortune...a cookie!* I've learned a secret...Chinese food is just a combination of protein, starch, veggies, and oil. Since I've learned how to choose it, I've also learned how to behave.

Portion control is the whole nine yards. However, learning portion control in this country is not easy. One day, I approached my nephew and asked him, "Stan, how much chicken do you think is a normal portion?" He quickly responded, "I guess about a bucket full." I chuckled. He was right. I used to put the bucket on the table and when it was empty, I was full.

For years, I carried a piece of diet cake to dinner parties so I could eat dessert. I feel so foolish, now. What could I have actually imagined was in that box that could possibly have made that cake diet?

When I think about it, I laugh at the prospect that I could have thought they made that cake from flour grown in diet wheat fields, eggs laid by diet chickens, or milk given by diet cows. I was stupid not to realize it was simply a small portion of regular cake. Perhaps, they fooled me by putting the program equivalents on the back of the box—one protein, one starch, one oil, *one dog, one cat, one goldfish.* That made it look so official that it mislead me!

Sure, diet cake allowed me to stay on my program. What good did that do? It never taught me how to live in the real world or how to eat a real piece of cake. In fact, continuing to believe there truly was diet cake trapped me in the FAT WORLD. My diet brain enlarged the smallest indiscretion so much that even a tiny "forbidden" crumb made me suffer as much quilt as if I had eaten an entire Kentucky Fried Chicken franchise.

I don't need diet foods any more to help me control my portions. I carefully do that for myself. It's simple. I only put on my plate what I intend to eat—and only eat what is on my plate. And, I always do that in advance. I know that once I pick up my fork and start eating, I run the risk of developing *"amnesia"* and forgetting how much food is really an appropriate portion.

One afternoon, I was explaining the food choices to a new member. For someone who had spent her entire life on a diet, she asked me a very legitimate question. "What spoon do I use to measure a teaspoon full of something? A regular spoon from my flatware set or a measuring spoon?" That poor lady worried that the wrong teaspoon full of something would make her FAT.

Can't blame her. Years back, I was on a diet that required that I eat three beef meals weekly. I dreaded it as I don't like beef very much. Yet, it was the requirement, so I felt I had to do it. Perhaps, if I could have had a little bit of ketchup, it would have made a big difference. My luck, ketchup was a "no-no," so, of course, I didn't eat it. I was afraid that if I did, I would never lose weight. What the heck was I afraid of? Did ketchup make me FAT? I doubt it. THIN people eat ketchup!

When one of my members was planning a celebration for her husband's birthday, she told me, "I am going to order a diet ice cream cake for him." "That's nice," I said, "is that his favorite?" "Oh no," she responded, "he loves real cake. I can't have that, though, and I want to have dessert at the party."

"Real cake," I asked, "what's real cake in comparison to diet ice cream cake?" She looked puzzled. I continued, "How many calories are there in a piece of diet ice cream cake? In contrast, how many calories are there in a piece of real birthday cake?" She said, "I really don't know. I never thought about it. All I know is that one is "legal" and one is not."

I went further, "Suppose, roughly speaking, there were the same amount of calories in a slice of either cake. Which would you prefer?" Quickly she admitted, "I'd grab the real cake." I went on, "But, just suppose there were ten or twenty more calories in one or the other. Would that change your mind?" "Nope," she admitted. "And, what if you had to have a smaller slice of one than the other to make it equal? Would you still choose the diet cake?" She smiled and announced, "He's getting a real cake for his birthday!"

Knowing the caloric content of food is essential to making the right choices. So is sometimes eating the foods you enjoy, even if it necessitates having smaller portions. It's just as important to satisfy your appetite, as it is to satisfy your hunger.

There will always be some folks who insist that you cannot lose weight if you eat "forbidden" foods. Gads, I think I've heard that one a million times in the last few years. Since I eat **ALL** foods—and have lost a considerable amount of weight—it's easy to tell them they're wrong.

FOOD IS JUST FOOD and its function is to nourish our bodies and please our palates. Furthermore, food is not fattening. If it was...then everyone would be FAT!

Food is not a reward or punishment—a hiding place or a party. Food is not the antidote for depression, fatigue, loneliness, insecurity, or anger. Food is not feelings—joy, sorrow, fear, hurt, disappointment, or anxiety.

For years in diet class, I heard, "Just stay on the program ...stay on the program...stay on the program." Oh sure, that helped me produce many temporary weight losses, but I could never maintain them. Dieting never helped make me aware of the inappropriate ways that I used food. But, I never blamed the diets. I always blamed myself. I allowed my diet failures to make me feel that I wasn't smart enough, strong enough, or good enough to be THIN. I just accepted that the DIET WORLD was right about me...I was weak.

The feeling of "I am not good enough" resulted in total rejection of myself. My mind made a natural calculation— dieting should be enough—and I never made it on a diet. Elementary, I'm not good enough. I concluded that if I couldn't be "good" on a simple diet, I was stupid and unworthy.

Worst of all, I felt the only way I could ever prove that I was good enough was to lose weight. Yet, I couldn't sustain the willpower I needed to resist food because I had an "inner emptiness" that made me feel hungry inside. A binge was the mission to help fill up that emptiness and after the binge, I despised myself for my weakness. Do you recognize the all too familiar vicious cycle of dieting?

Of all the misery and shame I experienced during my life in the FAT WORLD, that self-condemnation was the most excruciating pain of all.

I believed the diet lie that I was powerless....powerless to control food...powerless to change my attitudes...and power-less to correct my behaviors. Ridiculous! The REAL truth

141

...food had no power—except the power that I gave it. Well, if I gave it power, I could take that power away. There is nothing wrong with me. It is the DIET WORLD that is wrong. I've got what I need to be THIN. I have the power. I've always had it! I am smart enough, strong enough, and good enough to be THIN. IT IS THE DIET WORLD THAT IS NOT ENOUGH.

When I was a child, I remember my dad telling me that if you see something that is wrong—and say nothing—you become part of that wrong. Well, Daddy, don't worry. I won't let that happen. For the rest of my life, I'm going to try to right the diet wrong...and prove that **FOOD IS JUST FOOD!**

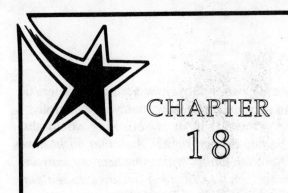

CHAPTER
18

WHAT'S IN THE ROAD...AHEAD?

I went kicking and screaming into my fight for control. I had a million excuses and two million alibis for my inability to stay on a diet. I blocked my own way by refusing to confront the truth. I felt I was unable to meet my own needs or solve my own problems effectively without food. I was out of touch with the "truth" about how to end my overeating and that prevented me from correcting the behaviors that caused it. One diet failure after another convinced me that no matter how hard I tried, I would never be able to succeed. I was living proof that it's impossible to do a positive thing in a negative atmosphere...

Every time I uttered the words, "I can't because"... I built a barrier that was impossible to cross. And brother, I had more hurdles to overcome than an Olympic jumper.

For starters, I forfeited the power to change my problems by refusing to assume responsibility for them. It was easier to blame my eating problems on circumstances beyond my control. For example, everyone in my family was overweight all the way back throughout history. Therefore, I excused my FAT as my destiny—my family heritage. Unfortunately, that defense didn't last long. As the result of a fluke, it was contradicted.

In addition to being overweight, it was also characteristic for the children in my family to have blue-eyes. Naturally, I always took it for granted that all my offspring would also have light eyes. Family history, right? *And, that might have happened if Paul Newman hadn't broken my heart by marrying Joanne Woodward. Until then, it never occurred to me that anything could alter that tradition.* But, believe me, when my Howie—and his big brown eyes—came along, offering me a deal too good to pass up, I grabbed it.

Our marriage led to Barbara having brown eyes, forever changing my family history. And, if that wasn't remarkable, I can't describe how amazing it is that Janet turned out to be a size five. *I swiftly retired family history as an excuse for my FAT.*

Okay, I lost that excuse. No big deal. I had a million more! I couldn't possibly be expected to stick to a diet when I hated veggies and fruit...*and loved chocolate.* When I was working, there was simply no time to cook. When I wasn't working, I had too much time on my hands, so I had to eat all day. And if I was sick—or anyone else in the world was sick—I couldn't diet.

In the summer, it was too hot—and in the winter, it was too cold! If I got a job or lost a job—if we took a trip or didn't have time to travel—no matter what, I found an alibi for not being responsible for my weight.

For sure, I needed food when I felt tired, nervous, anxious, rejected, frightened, angry, happy, sad, or anything else. If I got good news, bad news or NO news, I sealed my fate by uttering the words, "Well, I can't do it, so I might as well just give up and EAT."

Looking back, I can see that an enormous quantity of my overeating was done without my full awareness. Through a lifetime of repetition, some habits became part of my everyday life and I responded to food cues without even thinking.

In addition, I didn't realize that I had developed the *"YES, BUT"* syndrome. My responses became so automatic, I didn't even have to think before uttering them. If someone asked me if I wanted to be THIN, I'd snap back, *"YES, BUT*...what do you want from me? I've tried everything...every diet known to mankind. I've even had the shots from the placenta of a pregnant woman, accompanied by a five-hundred-calorie a day diet." *Tell me, if I could have stayed on a five-hundred-calorie diet, why did I need those shots?*

YES...I wanted to be THIN—*BUT*...I was just waiting for the right diet to come along...*hot dogs, french fries, and ice cream sundaes.*

If I had to choose the biggest obstacle in the way of my success, I'd say that it was that I never expected to be successful. In diet class, no matter how motivating or exciting the lecture, it was nullified by the fact that I had lost and regained the weight so many times, I didn't trust the program to lead me to success. When you have reservations about your ability to succeed—and expect to fail—there is no hope.

I kept going around in circles. I couldn't succeed by dieting, and I didn't have faith in myself to design a program that properly suited my needs. I held fast to my "diet mentality" because I lacked the information on how to find long-term gratification.

Of course, when I put all those hurdles in my path, little did I know that the day would come when I'd have to jump over them. Well, that day came.

I courageously began to expand my horizons beyond the programmed responses of the past. Having the courage to rely on myself and follow my own path—rather than playing

it safe by listening to the orders of the DIET WORLD—
helped me become self-reliant. So, good-bye roadblocks!

In the past, I didn't want to take responsibility for my
weight. I preferred to blame my environment, or the fates,
or the diets I had tried, or anything else I could think of...as
long as it was never my fault! In reality, it was probably a
combination of all those circumstances that caused my weight
problem. So what? I am still the person who is one-hundred
percent responsible for the solution!

A positive attitude can move mountains. Unfortunately,
my Howie doesn't have one. He has a tendency to be
negative—not the kind of dismissal that says, "you can't have
it," —the kind that says, "you can't do it." He can come up
with, at least, a thousand reasons why something won't work.
*One day, I got so frustrated that I bought him the book, The
Power of Positive Thinking. That was a big mistake. Now,
he's positive "it can't be done."*

However, if I persist, "Howie dear, if it could be done, how
would you do it?" He always comes up with an answer.
THIN is a matter of finding new solutions to old problems.

When I was on a plan requiring a real meal for breakfast
—fruit, starch and protein, I'd begin my morning by cheating.
I just couldn't eat all that food in the morning. *Well, if you
begin the day by cheating, trust me, you certainly don't improve
much as the day continues.* When I changed the rules for
breakfast, I eliminated any reason to cheat! I became a
problem solver...instead of a problem maker!

The THIN WEIGH was born to give us hope—to help us
focus on what we CAN do—and not dwell on what we
CAN'T eat. It is possible to eliminate the obstacles in our
path...by finding suitable methods to remove them. Hope is
a powerful way to overcome obstacles.

By removing the roadblocks, we can turn, "I can't" into

"who says I can't? I equate that moment to when Dorothy in the *Wizard of Oz* discovered that the power of the ruby slippers was simply believing that she could get home to Kansas. The power of our ruby slippers is the faith that we can be THIN.

Believing in yourself can propel you forward and self-confidence can allow you to take control of your own destiny. A good self-esteem and a feeling of worthiness is the guarantee that no one—or nothing—could stop you from achieving your goal. You've gotta believe! You are your best hope for the future. *Do you suppose Babe Ruth would have ever hit his first home run, if he hadn't believed that he could play baseball, and had taken up bowling instead?*

I know that nothing can block my path to success except me. Only the decisions that I make for myself can determine what I will accomplish in my life.

For the first time in my life, I began to value what I was *gaining* instead of what I was *losing*. I stopped worrying about why I couldn't eat as much as I wanted and got excited about being able to eat anything I wanted in portion control ...and still lose weight.

Weight wasn't all that I was losing. Sure, I was saying "so long" to overeating, but I was also saying "good-bye" to hating myself...guilt...diet failures...shame...and despair.

Control is the key, but it was not always easy to differentiate between what I could control and what was not mine for controlling. I suffered a lot of grief in my lifetime trying to manage matters that were beyond my control. True, I can choose for myself, but only for myself. Now, I've stopped wasting my energy trying to fix things that are outside of my domain.

I started my journey to the THIN WORLD because my Howie had ten pounds to lose. We've had many battles because I tried to force him to control himself to discard the weight, but for naught. I've lost my weight and NOW he has twelve pounds to lose. Truth is, I can only control myself—no one can control me—and I can't control anyone else.

Howie does have an explanation for his lack of success, however. When his doctor reminded him that he still hadn't lost weight, he told him, "I just can't get motivated." *Believe me, I spent the rest of the day reminding Howie of my life's work.* Sure it hurts me, but he is absolutely right. He said, "I can't," and that settled that.

I think I'll buy him a copy of the children's story, *The Little Engine That Could.* Remember that wonderful tale of the little train climbing the mountain, huffing and puffing and saying, "I think I can...I think I can...I think I can..."

I'm not going to try to fool you by telling you that changing is a snap. It's tough to diminish a compulsive activity, but it can be replaced by learning to embrace a positive outlook on life.

We can cease blaming the fates for our lot in life. We can stop trying to control everything. We can accept ourselves and others as we really are. We can look to ourselves for fulfillment—instead of to food to fill us up. We can do for ourselves what we have always asked food to do for us. Although, we cannot change the past—we can choose not to relive it.

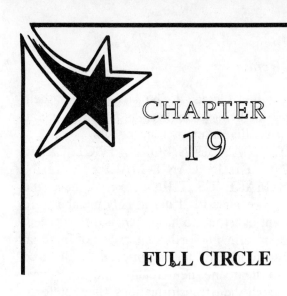

CHAPTER
19

FULL CIRCLE

I began by wishing on a star to be THIN. Now, I have not only become THIN...I have finally defined it...

THIN is no longer a number on a scale taken from an insurance chart...no longer a matter of my dress size. I consider my body only the house I live in—and I am the occupant inside. I will never again judge—or allow anyone else to judge me by my looks—as only what I AM is important. THIN gave me a new sense of self, a pride in who and what I am. By having the courage to take the responsibility for my own choices, I rid myself of the restrictions imposed upon me by dieting. I developed the faith and the courage to accept myself with my strengths and weaknesses, shedding the unrealistic expectation of perfection. I have no need to look to food as a means of enjoying my life, or for comfort in my times of sorrow. I now handle that for myself.

THIN has new meaning to me...THIN is simply knowing, loving, trusting, and controlling myself. THIN is me...and...I am THIN!

I have lost my weight and developed a THIN LIFESTYLE. I have ended my suffering, my shame, and my despair. In addition, many of my members are also triumphing. Yet, even though, others are using my story to become THIN, I am not satisfied. I feel blessed to be able to help them escape the sentence of living their lives as prisoners in the DIET WORLD. But, that alone is not enough.

A NEW REALITY HAS BEEN BORN. FOOD CAN'T MAKE US THIN. DIETS CAN'T MAKE US THIN. ONLY WE CAN MAKE US THIN. We all have the power, if we believe we have it! I did it. My members are doing it. Now, I want everyone to have a chance to succeed.

In my classes, we are bringing forth a new wave of freedom ...freedom to choose food. My life is enriched by all those who have come to hear the new reality and who have accepted it. As I watch their transformations, they reinforce my hope that someday we would all be free.

There are so many stories that I will never be able to mention them all. For as long as I live, however, I will remember the wonderful "before and after faces" of my THIN WEIGH family!

It started with Paula...MY FIRST STAR. (*A STAR is a THIN WEIGH member, who has reached his or her ideal weight.*) She was enthusiastic from day one, exclaiming, "This is for me," when she saw the treats. I'm not sure which one of us was more excited when she reached her ideal weight— me or Paula? After I pinned the STAR on her shoulder, she became my first part-time employee...my only part-time employee. Although the classes were going well for those who attended, getting members was very difficult. The business was having a tough time because there was so much competition. I was afraid that I could not fight the newspapers filled with ads bigger than any ads I could afford. I knew that I couldn't vie with the radio and television as they screamed claims of instant success. I didn't have the financial resources to compete in their league, so I looked for alternatives to keep the dream alive. Wonderful PAULA worked for peanuts...a *quarter of a cup equals one treat...* marketing the THIN WEIGH. She distributed flyers, arranged on-site classes, and beat the bushes for business to keep enough money in the till to continue.

Many times, when I felt worn out and defeated, it was Paula's energy that kept me going. The STAR I pinned on her shoulder never let me forget our mission.

Beautiful KATHY walked into a Wednesday night class with more than forty pounds to lose and walked out a STAR! It brought me pleasure to watch her melting each week. I especially cherish the moment when she first discovered that she could eat the foods she loved and still be THIN.

She worked in a beauty salon and through her success, many of her customers became members. They wanted to duplicate her effort, allowing her triumph to make a marvelous contribution to our cause.

Lovely ADRIENNE wanted to be THIN so badly. She was faithful—never missed a week—yet, her battle was tough. Food had such a strong hold on her that I often feared it was going to win. But she stubbornly refused to surrender.

A lifetime in diet classes had programmed her to believe that you were only good when you saw a smaller number on the scale, so she stopped weighing herself. She came to class three times a week, refusing to allow herself to become defeated.

To date, her struggle continues. She courageously and stubbornly refuses to believe that anything can prevent her from reaching her goal. Many times, her courage inspired me when it would have been much easier to give up then to continue fighting to keep the THIN WEIGH alive.

Parents, GLEN and JUDY, carried adorable KATRINA into class in an infant seat. They each had seventy-five or

more pounds to lose. They were looking for a better life
for their little one than the life FAT had provided them.
The very least they felt they owed their baby was healthy
parents—and a healthier attitude toward food. Together,
they have already lost well over one hundred pounds. What
they have "gained" can never be measured.

When ADELE walked into my class, recommended by one
of my other members, my first thought was, "What is she
doing here?" She certainly didn't have much weight to lose.
Then, I found out that was because she had spent her whole
life on a strict, strict, strict diet. When she heard there was
a place where no foods were "forbidden," she came to see if
that could possibly be true. It was tough going in the
beginning for her to select treats. Her diet training had
thoroughly programmed her to avoid them.

She slowly began to change. It began with pizza—Chinese
food followed—and then, one by one, she added other foods.
Week after week, I enjoyed watching her face show the look
of both wonder and delight as she experimented enjoying her
food and losing weight! Now, she can eat everything she can
control, and she is learning to control everything.

The day she became a STAR, she brought me a bag of my
beloved Hershey's Kisses with a pink bow on them. I loved
the candy, of course, but it was her note that I will never
forget. It simply said, "Thanks for the rest of my life." No
more needed to be said.

LESLIE didn't have too much weight to lose either, but
she was willing to make any sacrifice to get to her ideal
weight. When I mentioned the treats on the program, she
immediately rejected the idea of eating anything fattening.
She did admit to a fondness for cookies, though. I assured
her that she could include them, and still lose weight, but she
was skeptical. In an effort to convince her, I offered her a

free week if she ate the cookies and didn't lose any weight. She accepted that deal.

The following week, she assured me that she had made wonderful choices, except for the three cookies she had eaten. As she walked over to the scale, it was obvious that her knees were shaking. She was visibly nervous—positive that she was about to face disaster. Then, as the scale moved, she screamed with joy! She had eaten three cookies and lost three pounds!! Never again will she believe that you can get FAT from eating any food—in control.

Last, but not least is PHYLLIS. Perhaps, she best illustrates what the THIN WEIGH is all about. Before THIN WEIGH, she lost one hundred and ten pounds on another program and maintained it for fifteen years by strictly adhering to a diet code of ethics. However, she did not feel free...or comfortable with food...or with herself. She has spent the last two years fighting the battle for control.

She is finally aware that the issue is not food...or a weight loss. She's concentrating on learning how to take possession of her self and escaping the slavery of deprivation and bingeing. She is looking for victory and has set her sights on a better way of life. This time, she knows it isn't about the scale. This time, she knows it isn't about food. This time, she knows it's about PHILLY...and being herself. She has made a commitment to reclaiming her life. She has made slow and steady progress. She has made me very proud!

The list of STARS increased. Every time I awarded a STAR, my hope to see the light at the end of the tunnel grew. Not everyone lost weight immediately and instantly became a STAR. Some stayed in class for months and months—not losing weight, just fighting for control. They refused to give up, knowing that it takes some people longer to learn than others. They had heard the new message...and they believed it.

The impossible dream was becoming a reality and hope was growing inside me that we really could stop the pain, stop the guilt, stop the shame. Still, there was much work left to be done. For all those who came, there were still so many that had never heard our new truth. I wanted desperately to figure out how I could STOP THE DIET WORLD, SO EVERYONE COULD GET OFF! How could I bring forth the message to all the world that food had no power except the power we gave it...how?

True, I had learned it and I was teaching it to my members. But, that alone was not be enough to insure that no one ever again would have to suffer the failure of another diet. It would not guarantee that no one ever again would have to endure the pain of being FAT. It couldn't confirm that there would never be a need for anyone to purge to manipulate a number on a scale. I wanted to safeguard the future from the possibility that anyone ever again would have to starve and die because they felt they weren't good enough because they weren't THIN enough.

Was it possible to hope the message that food was not the issue could reach every corner of the earth? Could I dare to hope that someday everyone would know that we are all entitled to be the best we can be and that we have the right to do it our way? We can all be the STARS of our own lives.

My dream was that everyone could be THIN, but I feared it must surely be an IMPOSSIBLE DREAM. Then again, how could anything be impossible? Hadn't I just proven if you can dream it, you can do it?

I had come full circle. Once again, I had a wish—a mighty big wish—and so I looked to the heavens, to the first STAR...

*"I wish that no one ever again will
have to bear the pain of being FAT."*

I know the odds are against the chances of my wish coming true in my lifetime, but there is an old expression in sports —IT AIN'T OVER TILL THE FAT LADY SINGS.

I can't speak for any other FAT LADY—just for me—but I promise I am never, ever, ever going to give up fighting for this plague to be over—*no matter how long it takes, no matter how tough it is.*

I will never give up until everyone arrives at DESTINA-TION THIN for that will be the day when this FAT LADY SINGS...

PART

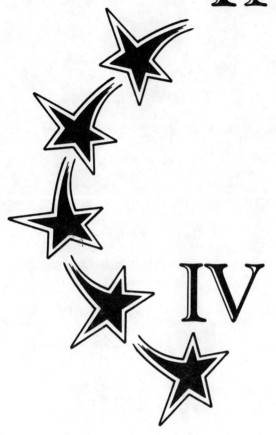

IV

THE
LIFESTYLER

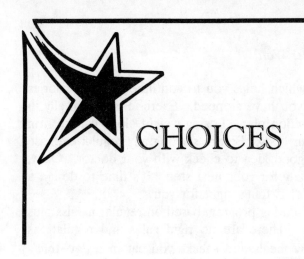

CHOICES

THE LIFESTYLER is not a magic formula for losing weight. It's not an easy way to take "control." It's not the guarantee of a THIN life. It's merely a guide to help you devise a healthy and enjoyable THIN LIFESTYLE.

Changing the way you have been eating all your life is certainly a major step. I congratulate you for having the courage to take action. The key to success lies in replacing negative habits and attitudes with a positive strategy.

When you plan your eating program keep in mind that variety, balance, and moderation are essential. Remember, too, that no matter how much you may like to ignore it—and regardless of what the great minds of the DIET WORLD say —the truth is that good nourishment must be your most important consideration.

Although it is outside of the scope of this book to give you a detailed course in nutrition, I heartily recommend that you seek other sources to obtain this vital information.

Once you have learned basic nutrition and positive behaviors, losing weight is really quite simple. *When you eat more calories than your body needs...you gain weight. When you take in fewer calories than you body needs...you lose weight.*

Another factor to consider is exercise. It is the best friend of anyone who wants to lose weight. Exercise not only burns up calories while you're doing it, but it also increases your metabolic rate which helps you to continue to burn calories for hours after you have stopped. Exercise is a vital ally in any weight reduction plan. Losing weight alone cannot firm and reshape your body. Before starting any regular exercise program, it's a good idea to check with your doctor. Okay, now you are ready for your next step. It's time to design a THIN LIFESTYLE that's right for you.

Organize your eating program based on regular meals...plus periodic snacks. There are no rigid rules and regulations about how many meals and snacks you eat in a day—that's your decision. However, once that decision has been made —after you have chosen an eating plan that suits your needs —follow it as consistently as possible. Eat the same amount of food at each meal and snack—at the same time every day —to teach your body positive eating habits...how to act THIN!

How many CHOICES each person needs in a day can vary with age, body size, and activity level. Therefore, you may want to consult your physician if you are uncertain as to exactly how many portions are right for you.

	Recommended Daily Choices		
	Minimum	Maximum	
WOMEN	13	15	Plus 500 Calories
MEN	15	18	a Week for Treats
YOUTH	15	18	

Of course, calories count—but not as much as you do! Neither man nor woman can live by bread alone—so, there is a "built in" allowance for you to use 500 calories a week... ANY WAY you want to! Naturally, it goes without saying that a calorie counter may be valuable. In the beginning, keep it simple. Don't start by trying to control something tough. Start with something easy—get success on your side— and then go forward from there.

The TREATS—just like ALL of your foods—should be eaten as part of your THIN LIFESTYLE. Plan to eat them in CONTROL. If you walk past a donut—stuff it into your face—and later decide to count it as a TREAT...you have controlled nothing! If you opt to enjoy dessert on Saturday night after dinner and eat a piece of cake or pie with your coffee—you're eating like a THIN person. Five hundred calories a week are YOURS to spend any way you want to ...so, ENJOY THEM!

To make it easy and flexible for you to make selections, THE LIFESTYLER is an exchange system of portions called CHOICES.

From the food lists that follow make your selections...and make it FUN. Finally, you have the freedom to eat the foods you LIKE...and skip the foods you DON'T LIKE. Believe me, there is no "one diet that fits all"...so create one that fits YOU!

Proteins

One CHOICE equals:
1 ounce (cooked)

BEEF	LIVER
CHEESE	LUNCH MEATS
CHICKEN	PORK
FISH	SHELLFISH
GAME	TURKEY
HOT DOGS	TURKEY COLD CUTS
LAMB	VEAL

One CHOICE equals:

COTTAGE CHEESE	1/3 CUP
EGG	1 MEDIUM
EGG SUBSTITUTES	1/4 CUP
EGG WHITES	2
FARMER CHEESE	1/3 CUP
RICOTTA CHEESE	1/4 CUP
TOFU	3 OUNCES

RECOMMENDED DAILY PORTION

MINIMUM: *3 choices*
MAXIMUM: *7 choices*

Dairy

One CHOICE equals:

BUTTERMILK . . . . 3/4 CUP
EVAPORATED SKIM . . . . 1/2 CUP
LO-CAL HOT COCOA . . . . 1 PACKET
LO-CAL MILKSHAKE . . . . 1 PACKET
LO-CAL PUDDING . . . . 1/2 CUP
NON-FAT DRY MILK . . . . 1/3 CUP
PUDDING POP 1
SKIM MILK . . . . 1 CUP
YOGURT, FROZEN . . . . 1/2 CUP
YOGURT, FRUITED . . . . 1/2 CUP
YOGURT, PLAIN . . . . 1 CUP

RECOMMENDED DAILY PORTION

MINIMUM: *2 choices*
MAXIMUM: *3 choices*

Extras

A 350 calorie frozen dinner = 4 CHOICES
A slice of plain or vegetable pizza = 3 CHOICES

Carbohydrates

One CHOICE equals:

BAGEL .... 1 OUNCE
BARLEY .... 1/2 CUP
BEANS .... 2 OUNCES
BEETS .... 1/2 CUP
BISCUIT .... 1 SMALL
BRAN FLAKES .... 1/2 CUP
BREAD .... 1 OUNCE
BREAD CRUMBS .... 3 TABLESPOONS
BREAD STICKS .... 2 (8 INCH)
CORN .... 1/2 CUP
CORN ON THE COB .... 1 SMALL
CORN OR WHEAT FLAKES ... 3/4 CUP
CORNBREAD .... 1 (2" SQ.)
COUSCOUS .... 1/2 CUP
CRISPBREAD .... 2 PIECES
ENGLISH MUFFIN 1/2
GRAHAM CRACKERS 2
GRANOLA .... 1/4 CUP
GRITS .... 1/2 CUP
LENTILS .... 1/2 CUP
LIGHT BREAD .... 2 SLICES
MATZO .... 1/2 BOARD
MELBA TOAST .... 4 SLICES
OATMEAL .... 1/2 CUP
OYSTER CRACKERS 20

Carbohydrates

One CHOICE equals:

PASTA . . . . 1/2 CUP
PEAS . . . . 1/2 CUP
PITA POCKET . . . . 1 OUNCE
POPCORN (PLAIN) . . . . 2 CUPS
POTATO . . . . 1 SMALL
PUFFED OATS, CORN,
 WHEAT OR RICE . . . . 1 CUP
PUMPKIN . . . . 3/4 CUP
RICE . . . . 1/2 CUP
RICE CAKES 2
ROLLS . . . . 1 OUNCE
SALTINES 6
SODA CRACKERS 4
SWEET POTATO . . . . 1/2 SMALL
TORTILLA OR TACO SHELL . . 1
WHEAT GERM . . . . 1/4 CUP
WINTER SQUASH . . . . 1/2 CUP

RECOMMENDED DAILY PORTIONS

MINIMUM: *3 choices*
MAXIMUM: *7 choices*

Fruits and Juices

1/2 CHOICE equals:

APPLE	1 SMALL
APPLE JUICE	1/3 CUP
APPLESAUCE (SUGAR FREE)	1/2 CUP
APRICOTS (DRIED)	4 HALVES
APRICOTS (FRESH)	2 MEDIUM
BANANA	1/2 MEDIUM
BERRIES	1/2 CUP
CANTALOUPE	1/2 SMALL
CHERRIES	12 MEDIUM
CIDER	1/3 CUP
CRANBERRY JUICE	1/4 CUP
DATES	2
FIGS	1
FROZEN FRUIT ON A STICK	1
FRUIT PUNCH	1/4 CUP
FRUIT SALAD	1/2 CUP
GRAPE JUICE	1/4 CUP
GRAPEFRUIT	1/2 MEDIUM
GRAPEFRUIT JUICE	1/2 CUP
GRAPES	20 MEDIUM
HONEYDEW	1 CUP
KIWI	1 MEDIUM
MANGO	1/2 SMALL
NECTARINE	1 SMALL
ORANGE	1 SMALL
ORANGE JUICE	1/2 CUP

Fruits and Juices

1/2 CHOICE equals:

PAPAYA . . . . 1/2 CUP
PEACH . . . . 1 MEDIUM
PEAR . . . . 1 MEDIUM
PERSIMMON 1
PINEAPPLE . . . . 1/2 CUP
PINEAPPLE JUICE . . . . 1/3 CUP
PLUMS . . . . 2 MEDIUM
POMEGRANATE SEEDS . . . . . . 3/4 MEDIUM
PRUNE JUICE . . . . 1/3 CUP
PRUNES . . . . 2 MEDIUM
RAISINS . . . . 2 TABLESPOONS
RHUBARB (NO SUGAR) . . . . . . 3/4 CUP
STRAWBERRIES . . . . 1 CUP
TANGERINE . . . . 1 LARGE
WATERMELON . . . . 1 CUP

RECOMMENDED DAILY PORTION

MINIMUM: *2 choices*
MAXIMUM: *4 choices*

Fats

1/2 CHOICE equals:

AVOCADO	1/2 CUP
BUTTER	1 TEASPOON
CREAM	1 TABLESPOON
CREAM CHEESE	1 TABLESPOON
DIET MARGARINE	2 TEASPOONS
HALF & HALF	2 TABLESPOONS
MARGARINE	1 TEASPOON
MAYO DIET	1 TABLESPOON
MAYONNAISE	2 TEASPOONS
OIL	1 TEASPOON
OLIVES	5 SMALL
PEANUT BUTTER	1 TABLESPOON
SALAD DRESSING LIGHT	1 TABLESPOON
SALAD DRESSING REGULAR	2 TEASPOONS
SEEDS	1 TABLESPOON
SOUR CREAM	2 TABLESPOONS

RECOMMENDED DAILY PORTION

MINIMUM: *2 choices*
MAXIMUM: *4 choices*

Veggies

MAY BE CHOSEN IN REASONABLE AMOUNTS
IN ADDITION TO YOUR DAILY CHOICES

ARTICHOKE
ASPARAGUS
BAMBOO SHOOTS
BEAN SPROUTS
BROCCOLI
BRUSSELS SPROUTS
CABBAGE
CARROTS
CAULIFLOWER
CELERY
CHICORY
CHINESE CABBAGE
COLLARD GREENS
CUCUMBERS
EGGPLANT
ENDIVE
ESCAROLE
FENNEL
KOHLRABI
LEEKS
LETTUCE

MUSHROOMS
MUSTARD GREENS
OKRA
ONIONS
PARSNIP
PEPPERS
PICKLES
RADISH
RUTABAGA
SAUERKRAUT
SCALLIONS
SHALLOTS
SNOW PEAS
SPINACH
STRING BEANS
SUMMER SQUASH
TOMATO
TURNIP
WATERCRESS
ZUCCHINI

RECOMMENDED DAILY PORTION
MINIMUM: 1/2 CUP

Goodies

*MAY BE CHOSEN IN REASONABLE AMOUNTS
IN ADDITION TO YOUR DAILY CHOICES*

BACON BITS . . . . 1 TEASPOON
BARBECUE SAUCE . . . . 1 TABLESPOON
BOUILLON . . . . 1 PACKET
CHILI SAUCE . . . . 1 TABLESPOON
CHOCOLATE SYRUP . . . . 1/2 TEASPOON
CORNMEAL . . . . 1 TEASPOON
CORNSTARCH . . . . 1 TEASPOON
FLOUR . . . . 1 TEASPOON
HONEY . . . . 2 TEASPOONS
JAM . . . . 1 TEASPOON
JELLY . . . . 1 TEASPOON
KETCHUP . . . . 2 TEASPOONS
MAPLE SYRUP . . . . 1 TEASPOON
MOLASSES . . . . 1 TEASPOON
NON-DAIRY CREAMER . . . . . . 1 TEASPOON
PANCAKE SYRUP . . . . 1/2 TEASPOON
PARMESAN CHEESE . . . . 1 TEASPOON
RELISH . . . . 1 TEASPOON
STEAK SAUCE . . . . 2 TEASPOONS
SUGAR . . . . 1 TEASPOON
TAPIOCA . . . . 1 TEASPOON
TARTER SAUCE . . . . 1 TABLESPOON
WHIPPED TOPPING . . . . 1 TABLESPOON

Freebies

*MAY BE CHOSEN IN REASONABLE AMOUNTS
IN ADDITION TO YOUR DAILY CHOICES*

BAKING POWDER
BAKING SODA
COFFEE
DIET BROWN SUGAR
DIET JELLY
DIET SALAD DRESSING (10 CALORIES)
DIET SODA
EXTRACTS
FLAVORINGS
HERBS
HORSERADISH
LEMON JUICE
MUSTARD
NON-STICK SPRAY
SOY SAUCE
SPICES
SUGAR FREE GELATIN
SUGAR FREE POWDERED DRINK MIXES
SUGAR SUBSTITUTE
TEA
UNSWEETENED COCOA
VINEGAR
WORCESTERSHIRE SAUCE

Recommendations:

1. Eat slowly and consciously.

2. Note the recommended daily portion for each food group.

3. Drink eight glasses of water a day.

4. Remove all visible skins and fats from foods before eating.

5. Avoid foods high in sodium.

6. Weigh and measure foods after cooking.

7. Read the labels on all foods.

8. Avoid eating between meals or snacks.

9. Prepare foods by broiling, baking, or roasting without additional fats.

10. Select skim or 1% dairy products.

11. Select skim or 1% cheese products.

PART

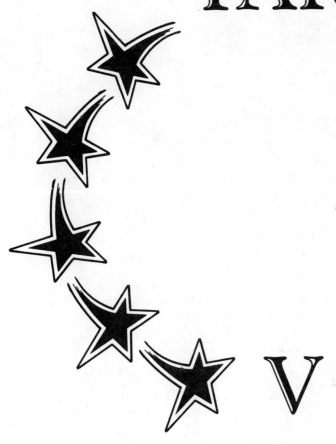

V

THE
END OF
THE TUNNEL

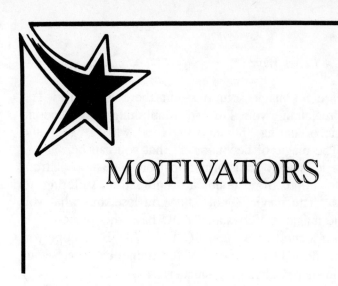

MOTIVATORS

Our journey is almost over. I hope that you have enjoyed the trip, thus far. Unfortunately, this is where I have to leave you and you'll be going it alone from here. Luckily, you don't have that much farther to travel as you are entering the final phase of your voyage. There's just one more stretch between you and the finish line.

On the pages that follow are fifty-two weekly motivators. They has been written to provide you with inspiration while you build the necessary skills to make a permanent lifestyle change.

THIN IS TRULY WITHIN YOUR REACH, so please fight hard to win the war over food. Your victory can make a valuable contribution to wiping out the vicious cycle of starving and overeating.

When you reach your ideal weight—without dieting—you confirm the theory that DIET IS A 4 LETTER WORD. When you end your deprivation, you intensify the truth that food is just food. As you learn to love yourself more than you love food, you fortify the conviction that THIN lies in the attitude. By not giving in to a "quick fix," you reinforce the reality that a permanent solution is available.

There are no magic solutions—but there is magic. The magic of reclaiming your life and establishing your freedom. The magic of eating and enjoying food without guilt and shame. The magic of becoming all that you can be.

The magic is your transformation from pain to joy...from despair to hope...from doubt to faith...from suffering to happiness. The magic is not what you lose...but what you gain! The magic is YOU...and YOU have the magic.

It's time for me to wish you BON VOYAGE. I hope you will follow the light at the end of the tunnel and reach your destination—happy...healthy...and...THIN.

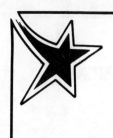

I BELIEVE!

I BELIEVE that dieting will never bring me the results that I seek. I BELIEVE that I can learn to listen to my body and its hunger signals. I BELIEVE that I can stop eating compulsively. I BELIEVE that I can trust myself and that I no longer need a step-by-step diet plan to handle my eating. I BELIEVE the pain of FAT is worse than the fear of change. I BELIEVE that change comes from taking risks and going a step further than I've ever gone before. I BELIEVE that I can cope with my life without a food crutch.

I BELIEVE that I have inner resources and the ability to overcome the compulsion to overeat. I BELIEVE that I deserve love and respect. I BELIEVE that I can love myself more than I love my food. I BELIEVE that life can offer peace and joy. I BELIEVE that I deserve to be happy. I BELIEVE that I can bury the past and all of the mistakes I made there. I BELIEVE that I can meet my needs directly. I BELIEVE that I—and I alone—am responsible for myself.

I BELIEVE that I have the power to control my life. I BELIEVE I can honor the commitment I made to live a THIN LIFESTYLE. I BELIEVE that I can say "no" to food and "yes" to life!

YOU BETTER BELIEVE IT!

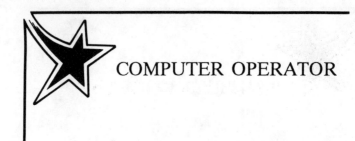

COMPUTER OPERATOR

The computer industry has certainly revolutionized the world. These days, computers control everything. What's the big deal? We humans have always been directed by a computer—the greatest computer ever devised—the human brain.

Your brain has the power to remember everything that it has ever been told. It has the ability to learn and relearn—to act and react—to respond and change responses. It has so much power that in your lifetime, you can never use your brain to its fullest potential.

Your sub-conscious mind is your brain's software. Unfortunately, it can only function as it has been programmed—and you have been programmed with "diet" software. Dieting never works...so erase your diet software. It is time to upgrade your approach to being THIN because new information is available.

You, as the operator of your computer, can develop new and improved behaviors with regard to losing weight. Override the outdated and old-fashioned diet myths of the past and replace them with new modern day thinking. Put THIN in your mind and soon it will spread to your waistline.

There is nothing that you can't do if you let your mind create a positive strategy for success. If you change your mind, you will change your life.

Sorry IBM, the world's most perfect computer is the brain!

THIN SOFTWARE, PLEASE!

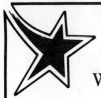

WHO DO YOU TRUST?

What do you think of yourself? Do you feel confident when making choices or do you need the reassurance of others before making a decision?

The contradiction between your ideals and the way you behave is the measure of your self-esteem. If you always follow the instructions of others, rather than trusting your own judgement, your level of self-esteem is low.

The world of dieting requires that you follow orders even if they don't suit you and your lifestyle. You had no choices!

Now, the idea is to bring your opinions, attitudes and judgements into line with the lifestyle that you want for yourself. Begin now and act like the person that YOU want to be. Trust yourself to design an eating style that suits you. Trust yourself to select the foods that you want to eat. Trust your body signals...eat when you are hungry and stop when you are full. Trust yourself to make the decisions that effect your life.

Make a realistic assessment of your strengths and weaknesses...your abilities and faults...your goals...and what you'd like to accomplish in your life. Approach life with optimism, but be realistic. Trust yourself and aim high. If you fall short, try again! Have faith in yourself. You have everything you need to become YOU.

TRUST YOURSELF!

LOOKING GOOD!

Are you starting to look THIN? Are you surprised when you see your reflection in a mirror...or catch a glimpse of yourself in a store window as you pass by? Is it tough for you to get used to being a new person?

Sure, you have made a change for the better...but, it's still a change...and change is not easy. People may respond to you differently or your own reaction to yourself may seem peculiar.

Be careful about your expectations for your THIN life. Getting THIN is not the guarantee of an automatic "happy" life. You may become more social. You may learn to play tennis. You may seek a new career. But, it is not losing weight that will turn your life around...it's you!

Life as a THIN person won't be one long party. Living in a complex world is tough. In the past, you had your "food crutch" to help you cope or your excess weight for an excuse to avoid facing difficult situations.

Well, it's time to re-enter the real world. Now you are on your own to make a new beginning. You have a new THIN body, inner peace, self-confidence, and a positive attitude. Looking good and feeling good about yourself... a wonderful start to living... really living. Enjoy yourself and have fun!

FEEL GOOD ABOUT LIFE

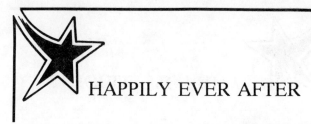# HAPPILY EVER AFTER

Have you spent your life on the vicious cycle of losing and gaining weight? Well, if you want a permanent solution to being overweight, a few basic changes must be made in your master plan.

Fad diets that promise FAST and EASY weight losses have been around throughout all eternity, but they must now be replaced by reasonable and realistic goals.

It may be necessary for you to change the people, places and things from your past in favor of a new, positive attitude focused on success.

The desire to overeat is an emotional and not a physical need. Therefore, it is important that you surround yourself with people who will reinforce your desire to reach your goal...and it is vital that you ask for their support!

By setting realistic goals...you can achieve success. By respecting and forgiving yourself for mistakes, you can avoid guilt. Your value as a person is not measured by how much you weigh. By learning to control the foods you love, you can escape deprivation. From the depths of uncontrollable overeating, you can rise up to find peace and happiness.

Deprivation, bingeing, and guilt lead to a low self-esteem which produces an empty feeling that no amount of food can satisfy. Fill yourself up with self-respect and inner peace and you will never be hungry again. Believing in yourself and trusting your ability to make your own choices is the path to being THIN.

BE THIN AND HAPPY!

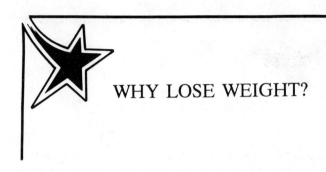

WHY LOSE WEIGHT?

I WANT TO LOSE WEIGHT BECAUSE...that special person in my life wants me to be thinner. It is bathing suit time and I want to look great at the beach. It's my Monday morning routine. It's much healthier and I owe it to my family. Everyone is nagging me and I want them to stop. My cousin is getting married and I want to look great at the wedding. Maybe, I can get a better job. I just can't stand myself.

For these reasons, you are willing to suffer through another dreary diet to lose weight. But, the chances for your success are not good...in fact, they are next to nil. There is only one reason to lose weight—because you want to become a THIN person—and you want to stay that way for the rest of your life.

If you are willing to take the responsibility for learning a new way of life—to reprogram your thinking of the past—to practice self-discipline—success will be yours.

Never again will it be necessary for you to suffer through another diet. Never again will you have to live with the shame and disappointment of failing. Never again will you have to punish yourself because you did not succeed. This time, lose weight for the right reason. Do it for yourself!

I'M DOING IT FOR ME!

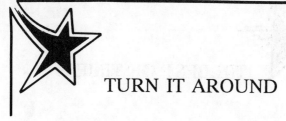

TURN IT AROUND

It's tough to win the war over food and it's impossible without the proper ammunition. Binge eating is both unplanned and uncontrolled as it is a response to feelings of relaxation, boredom, stress, loneliness, fear, etc.

Your attitude toward food was developed from your experiences. If, in the past, food was associated with warmth and security—or used to soothe pain—or as a reward for work well done—or as a symbol of love and friendship—it can become a natural reflex to turn to food in times of stress or joy.

In reality, food is only the fuel that keeps your body running. As you begin to control your feelings, you can begin to control your food. Food is not the center of your life or your life saver.

Sure, bingeing may have given you a temporary sense of exhilaration, but how long did it last? The delicious taste of the foods you love can bring you momentary pleasure, but for how long? It is always followed by a backlash of guilt, anguish, and more bingeing. It becomes a vicious cycle that can only be broken by eliminating the need to binge.

Binge eating cannot solve your problems. Learning to meet your needs directly—developing a good self-image—and keeping a positive attitude toward your ability to cope with your life—is the key. Believe in your own worth and see the value in yourself. You —not food—are the most important thing in your life.

BE YOUR BEST!

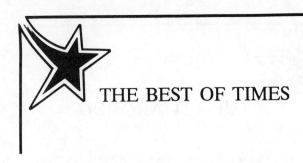

THE BEST OF TIMES

Today is not a dress rehearsal for tomorrow. Today is twenty-four hours of precious time. It is available to spend only once...so, don't waste it.

Yes, you have a history of dieting failure. No, you can't predict the future—but, you can live today to it's fullest. You can have the body that you've always wanted. You can live the life that you've always desired. You can experience joy. You can make wise choices and the right decisions for yourself.

In the past, perhaps you've filled your life with "maybe" —"but"—and "if only." Now, you are ready to take charge. There is no need to limit yourself to the past. Living is a challenge. Don't just let it happen...make it happen...your way.

It's foolish to spend time crying over what you can't do...can't have...or can't find. Maybe, yesterday was not satisfying—make today work for you—and who knows about tomorrow? There is no reason to wait for life to happen—because while you are waiting—life will be happening without you.

You are living a positive new lifestyle—not agonizing your way through another dreary diet. Make each day fun. The best time to take charge of your life is NOW.

Today is the only day that counts! Make this the best of times...time to get THIN...and stay THIN!

THE BEST OF TIMES IS NOW!

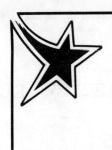

ONLY YOU

If being a THIN person is your destination, then chart a course to lead you to...a THIN LIFESTYLE. ONLY YOU know what route you want to travel.

On your trip, you may encounter a few unforeseen curves in the road. Simply adjust your map to handle these detours instead of allowing them to become a permanent change of direction.

Road blocks can prevent you from reaching your ultimate destination—so beware of building them. Stop blocking your mind. Don't tell yourself, "I can't ...I eat out too much. I can't...I love food. I can't... I'm weak." Tell yourself, "Yes, I can...if I say I can."

The road to your dreams must be honestly perceived and executed. Beware of the search for "quick-fixes" as they will rob you of the chance to find a long-term solution. Sure, the trip is long...it's tough ...and it's not always exciting, but you can do it. Tie your best information from the past to your best judgement for the future and create the best life that you can imagine for yourself.

ONLY YOU know the person inside of you. ONLY YOU can dream for yourself. ONLY YOU can make those dreams come true. So, will it be a road map or a road block? Will it be the journey to your ideal weight...or a lifetime of starving and bingeing? ONLY YOU can decide.

ONLY YOU CAN DO IT!

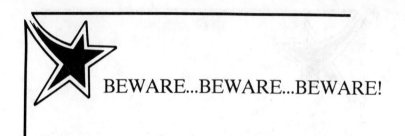

BEWARE...BEWARE...BEWARE!

As a result of spending much of your life as an overweight person, you may have certain conditioned reactions to sights, smells, and situations. The passage of time will certainly make these food cues lessen, however, the quickest way to change these reactions is to stop reinforcing them.

The presence of "trigger" foods, places associated with food, negative moods, positive moods, memories of the past, aromas, etc., make it tough to resist temptation.

Intentionally exposing yourself to difficult situations at difficult times is counter-productive. The best way to win the battle against desire is to be smart...not to be strong.

When you feel a powerful craving and want to prevent a binge, the objective is to handle the situation and survive.

It's not always necessary to "just say no." Often, it is better to satisfy the craving. If you want a piece of candy...eat it. It's better to eat a piece of candy... in control—then a bag of candy...out of control.

Sure, the past can "trigger" a reaction in the present, but you can stop it...by choosing to ignore it. A desire to overeat need not be a signal to overeat. Develop a new strategy to handle the old habits of the past.

TRIGGER SUCCESS!

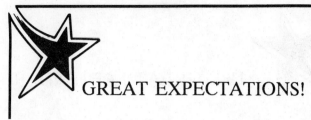

GREAT EXPECTATIONS!

Newspaper, television, and radio ads promising FAST AND EASY weight losses are endless. Well, don't believe them! Unrealistic goals lead to unhappiness because when a goal is unattainable—the failure is guaranteed. You judge what you have accomplished in contrast to what you have been promised—ending up tense—constantly demanding more and more of yourself—making it harder and harder to deliver results!

By setting simple goals and backing them up with hard work, you choose success...rather than setting up failure! There is no short-cut to changing the habits, attitudes, and beliefs of a lifetime. To change your eating style permanently, you have to practice your new habits over and over again, until they replace your old negative behaviors. Instead of short-term perfection, concentrate on making slow and steady progress.

Sure, you want to lose weight FAST...and you probably have many times...only to gain it back even FASTER... chalking up yet another failure. Losing weight is not enough unless it is combined with permanent lifestyle changes. Design a new master plan for a life filled with confidence, inner peace, and the resources to cope with daily living.

Lighten up and take life as it comes...satisfied with what you are accomplishing—correcting your mistakes —and living like a THIN person.

Don't set yourself up for failure because your expectations are too great...and you'll never be disappointed again!

EXPECT TO BE THIN FOREVER

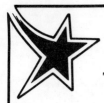

THE GREAT PRETENDER

Have you always wanted to be THIN? Well, what is holding you back? You can succeed...or you can make excuses for your lack of success. The choice is yours!

Be completely honest with yourself: How much do you want to be THIN? Enough to be THIN?

Is this you? I want to be THIN...but I don't have time to cook. I want to be THIN...but it's tough to change my eating habits. I want to be THIN...but I'm not ready to take control because my life is in shambles. I want to be THIN...but it's tough.

Sure, there can always be excuses to prevent you from reaching your goals in life, but can you think of one really good reason? Can you think of any other area of your life where you have as many alibis for your behavior as with your weight? You can solve your problems, if you search for honesty. Throw away your alibis and excuses and instead take responsibility for yourself.

So, think again about your desire to be THIN—and take another look at the excuses that you have been making to prevent it from happening. Stop lying to yourself. Stop pretending that you are doing your best. Stop telling yourself that you are not good enough to do the task at hand. YOU hold your future in your hands.

STOP PRETENDING...

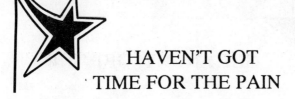

HAVEN'T GOT
TIME FOR THE PAIN

Life is to be lived...to be enjoyed...to be celebrated! But, sometimes we forget to hear the music—to smell the flowers—or to laugh. Instead, we view ourselves as victims because we are overweight in a world that worships THIN.

A victim is one who has no control over his or her destiny. A victim has no opportunity to make choices. YOU HAVE A CHOICE. You can regain control of your life. You can end the pain of being overweight.

For years, food may have beaten you, but now you can choose to stop the pattern of bingeing or starving. You can choose to end the pain of failure—choose to take control—choose to live a THIN LIFESTYLE.

This time is different. This time you have chosen to stop the pain...forever! You must address your feelings in control—address others in control—address your food in control. Live your life...your way!

Make your own choices. Pleasing others is not an appropriate reason to eat. Accepting food you don't want because you are uncomfortable to decline it only keeps you FAT. Tell a hostess, "thanks...but no thanks." Tell a loved one that positive reenforcement is what you need. Tell a "buttinsky" to mind his own business. Tell the whole world that you are in charge of calling your own shots. Live a pain free existence ...in control!

LIVE PAIN FREE

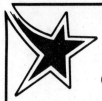

GET ANGRY, GET THIN!

Anger is often the cause of overeating—more so, than any other emotion. Anger—especially if it is repressed—can make you feel very uncomfortable and this discomfort can be confused with hunger.

In childhood, often parents unintentionally teach children how to repress anger. "It's not nice to get angry and lose your temper." "It's easier to catch flies with honey...so be sweet." You can run into trouble when you try to ignore feelings of anger as if they don't or shouldn't exist. Anger is a normal and natural feeling and it's okay to express it.

As your self-esteem rises and your confidence grows, you will be able to declare your anger more freely. In the meantime, take care not to bottle up your resentment until the pressure rises to an explosion level. Handle your wrath immediately. Direct it toward the real problem and avoid turning it toward yourself...with a binge.

Have you ever had a binge because you have been angry at someone? Well, you punished the innocent party. Don't let your anger at someone else trap you into overeating. Anger is not bad. It is a natural response to a situation where you feel you have been wronged. It's a way of saying, "Don't push me around." Anger expressed appropriately passes swiftly. Give yourself permission to express your anger.

GET ANGRY AT FAT!

I'M JUST TERRIFIC

Has your weight problem been a shield to avoid dealing with other aspects of your life? Do you use your weight as an excuse for not trying to achieve? Do you promise yourself that you will start living after you've lost weight? "If only I was thinner, I could handle my problems, I could realize my dreams ...if only I was thinner."

The thought of becoming THIN can be a bit scary, but, face that fear and do it anyway. Thinner, you may reach all your goals. Life is to be lived...so, go for it! You may make all your dreams come true— or maybe not— but, either way, you will be living life to the fullest—not letting your weight serve as a hiding place to avoid facing your fears.

Perhaps, in the past you were hiding the guilty secret of overeating, cheating, and sneaking. Well, that's all behind you, so come out from behind your "food hiding place."

Today, you can choose a different path...freedom. You can look good, feel good, be healthy. Your success or failure in life does not depend on what you eat—but rather on the decisions that you make for yourself. Begin living your life happily NOW. Looking good and feeling good about yourself—what a perfect duo! You are what you are...and that's just terrific!

CHOOSE LIFE AND LIVE IT!

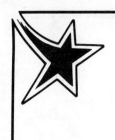

IT TAKES GUTS....

Losing weight, at best, is no fun. You can opt for the route of drinking liquids, eating diet cookies, pre-packaged foods, or any number of crash diets. They will all produce the desired results—if all you seek is a FAST weight loss. However, if you want a permanent solution, you have a more difficult task. It will take guts to make the changes to be THIN forever.

THIN people do not diet or starve—that's what FAT people do. THIN people eat and live—in control. You have chosen to live without a "food crutch" and that takes guts. You have chosen to win the war over food—and that takes guts. You have chosen to stop seeking "quick-fixes" in favor of long-term solutions—and that takes guts.

You are learning new and positive behaviors—and that takes guts. You are seeking solutions to your problems that don't include overeating—and that takes guts. It take real guts to face the enemy—and beat it—rather than just hiding away from it.

You'll need courage to hang in there and fight. When the going gets tough—it takes guts to get tougher. But one day, you are going to reach your ideal weight—and no longer need guts. Living like a THIN person doesn't take guts!

GIVE 'EM HELL

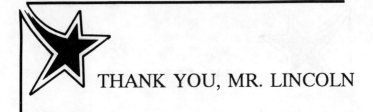

THANK YOU, MR. LINCOLN

Abraham Lincoln is best known for freeing the slaves and leading this country through a bitter civil war. Have you ever known freedom...or have you only known the bitterness of serving two masters... FOOD and DIETS?

Want freedom? Then fight your personal civil war and seize emancipation. The struggle for freedom is not easy. It demands great sacrifice and dedication to purpose and there are no guarantees.

On the day Lincoln issued the Emancipation Proclamation, the slaves were not granted freedom. They were only given the right to be free. Much work was still left to be done. You, too, have declared your desire to be emancipated from dieting, bingeing and slavery...but, still there is much to be done.

War is difficult...but victory is sweet. When your battle has been won, you will never again have to face life as a slave. You will be free to live the life that you have always yearned for—a life in CONTROL.

You owe it to yourself to be free to be the best you can be. You are not a slave. You can escape. Not quite free yet, but so what? You may not be exactly what you want to be, but you have made a firm beginning... so rejoice. After all, you are not what you used to be.

It takes courage to win the war...but, you have everything you need to be everything you want to be.

HONEST ABE, I WANT TO BE FREE

THE MOUSE TRAP

A delicious looking piece of cheese sitting atop a block of wood with a hidden metal spring can look very attractive. But, once invaded—GOTCH YA!

The promise of a FAST AND EASY weight loss is like a piece of cheese—luring YOU to see just what you want to see—hear only what you want to hear—and believe only what you want to believe...GOTCH YA!

Sure, you see ads that promise EASY weight losses. You hear words promising that you can lose weight FAST. If you are suckered into believing that you are not responsible for doing the hard work that will lead you to success...GOTCH YA!

Of course, it's tempting to accept the EASY way—to follow the crowd—to do what is fashionable—to throw yourself into a short-term commitment hoping to solve your long-term problems. But, is it worth it when this cycle leads only to frustration, despair, unhappiness and...GOTCH YA!

The problem of being overweight cannot be solved by reaching for a tempting piece of cheese. A permanent solution lies in the determination and motivation to change. If you don't alter the present, you will be doomed to repeat the mistakes of the past, and become trapped forever in the FAT WORLD.

Make a commitment to change old habits and eating behaviors. Fight the war over food...and WIN. It's your turn to say to the DIET WORLD—GOTCH YA!

I WON'T BE TRAPPED...

WELCOME
TO FANTASY ISLAND!

Do you fantasize about what it would be like to eat anything you want...just like THIN people? Can you imagine how it would feel to wear any style of clothes ...just because you like them...and not because they fit? Do you picture yourself acting like the life of the party and never again having to refuse an invitation because you are embarrassed about how you look? Fantasy? Why not reality?

It's time to leave FANTASY ISLAND and get to work making those dreams come true! It's time to live like a THIN person. Your life does not have to revolve around food. It's time to find new activities, new interests, new thoughts. It's time to walk down new avenues that don't lead to food...but to FUN!

Picture yourself taking charge of your life—getting to know yourself—and liking it. Come out from inside your overweight body and be YOU. You can chart your own course and measure even your smallest success as a milestone. Your positive attitude and a new THIN lifestyle will be your ticket to triumph.

THIN people can be your best example. They are proof that THIN is no fantasy! Make the decision to choose the reality of a brand new YOU...or spend the rest of your life waiting for the plane to take you to Fantasy Island.

MAKE YOUR FANTASY A REALITY

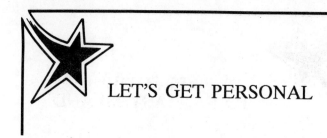

LET'S GET PERSONAL

The personal ad craze is sweeping the country. Classified ads are placed to sell old furniture, buy new goods, find a job, or quit one. Now advertisements are even being used in hopes of finding the perfect relationship.

Newspapers are also filled with ads trying to enlist participation in "fast weight loss" programs. What if the tables were turned? Have you ever wondered what an ad for the perfect diet would look like?

"FAT PERSON SEEKS DIET FOR LIFELONG RELATIONSHIP. MUST BE FAST, EASY, PERMANENT, AND RESPONSIBILITY FREE. NO FOODS MAY BE FORBIDDEN AND PORTIONS MAY NOT BE RESTRICTED. GUILT, SHAME, OR FAILURE CANNOT BE ALLOWED. NO CHANGE IN LIFESTYLE MAY BE REQUIRED. PROVISIONS MUST BE INCLUDED FOR FOOD TO BE USED FOR FUN, COMFORT, PROBLEM SOLVING, ENTERTAINMENT, LOVE, AND COMPANIONSHIP. RESULTS MUST BE GUARANTEED AND EFFORTLESS."

Who would answer an ad like that? Only someone who did not have the good sense to know there is no perfect diet. Diets do not make people THIN.

Let's get personal—do you really want to be THIN? THEN...BE THIN! To find success, you must be fully committed to learning to think, eat, and act in a new way. Your dream to be THIN must be stronger than your desire for a "quick fix". You can advertise for it, wait for it, or—better yet—work for it.

ADVERTISE THE NEW YOU!

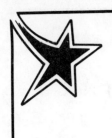

YOU'LL NEVER BE
THE SAME

For years, have you lived with the curse of being overweight...always searching for the next diet panacea? Why?

Each time you reach for pills, shots, powders, fad diets, you are reinforcing your ability to FAIL. Diets never worked—and even if they did—working was losing weight—only to gain it back. No wonder, you failed...you were looking in the wrong place for a solution.

Perhaps, once you thought that THIN was beyond your reach. But, now you know you have a future without limit. Today instead of letting your negative emotions direct your life, you can use your positive attitude to propel you forward.

You need not repeat the past. Your awareness is different now. NEVER AGAIN will you have to suffer on a diet. You have heard a new truth and you'll never be the same again. The word diet will never again have a positive meaning for you. You can never again deny that if you live and eat like a THIN person...you will be THIN!

Losing weight is no longer a yoke you have to wear. Instead, you can live each day in control—feeling entitled to your new thinner...happier self.

A new beginning...how fabulous! From this day forward...you'll never be the same again.

NEVER THE SAME AGAIN!

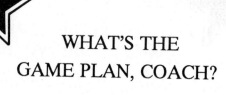

WHAT'S THE
GAME PLAN, COACH?

The coach of a football team develops a plan for winning the game. A director needs a script to direct a movie or play. An architect draws a plan for a contractor to build a house...

To be a THIN person, you have to be the architect, director and coach of your new THIN lifestyle!

Everyone is different—some folks choose to eat three meals each day—or a large breakfast and no lunch—or a large lunch and no breakfast. Maybe, some choose to eat dinner at 6:00 P.M. and some dine at midnight! No matter, if it suits your eating style—so, first step—the game plan.

When the plan has been drawn—the script written —the director takes action. Give yourself the proper guidance to make the choices that are included in your new lifestyle. Follow the script all the way to your ideal weight—even if you have to rehearse and rehearse until your performance is fully automatic and flawless!

The plan written and rehearsed—play the game. As the coach...it is your job to provide the motivation to do your very best. Be positive! Congratulate yourself on your wonderful game plan...encourage yourself to play your very best. YOU are a winner!

TOUCHDOWN!

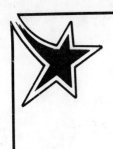

WHO CARES?

Sometimes it's tough to re-act to life's pressures. Many times we encounter thoughtless people or situations beyond our control. Makes you wonder if anyone cares?

Sure life can be tough—but so can you! If something goes wrong—don't give up—fix it. Even if the game is not going your way—play it anyway.

If you feel that life is lonely—and that the world around you doesn't care—don't stop caring! If you can't have everything that you want—want everything you can have.

It's difficult to be overweight in a THIN world. Sometimes fear of disapproval can lead to an "I don't care, anyway" attitude. The best way to overcome that attitude is to love yourself—for what you are— and not for how you look.

Sometimes being a THIN person gets confused with how the world is treating you. In truth, the real incentive for being a THIN person is because you care enough about yourself to be the best you can be.

Feeling entitled to success is one of the key ingredients in being successful. So, take care of yourself. Care enough to make a commitment to be THIN...then care enough to honor that commitment.

WHO CARES? I DO!

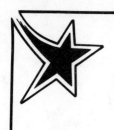

IF AT FIRST

Success begins first in the mind. Successful people have faith in their ability to achieve their goals. The perception that you can reach your goal—coupled with belief in yourself—combined with dedication of propose—ALWAYS leads to success.

However, allowing the judgement of others to assess your results and thereby preventing you from persevering will surely doom you to failure. Doubting yourself can become an insurmountable barrier to finding success. Instead believe that you can succeed and then slowly move forward a little bit at a time. Instant results do not guarantee permanent success.

You have the ability to be THIN, but first you must win the battle in your mind. Act like a THIN person and that is exactly what you will become. You need not be a slave to food...or remain a prisoner in the world of diets. Just make up your mind to be free.

If the scale doesn't give the results you want, don't quit. If your emotions get the best of you...don't quit. If others try to sabotage you...don't quit.

Have the patience to continue no matter how long it takes. You have the strength to deal with your problems, no matter how tough they are. See yourself as a winner and the fight is easier.

DON'T TRY...DO!

KEEP IT MOVING

There is no better friend to someone who wants to lose weight than exercise. Exercise is the best way to use up the energy your body stores in the form of extra pounds. Additionally, it burns calories and leads to total body fitness.

Exercise can improve cardiac function, reduce blood pressure, lower cholesterol and triglycerides...all reducing the risk of heart disease. Exercise can contribute to building stronger bones, thereby aiding in the prevention of osteoporosis. Exercise helps you increase your stamina. It can also lead to more restful sleep, which can help decrease depression or anxiety.

Best of all, regular exercise—at least, twenty minutes a day, three times a week—can effect your metabolic rate and help you lose weigh more efficiently. In addition, regular exercise is also critical to weight maintenance.

So, even though, you may not be a Jane Fonda or a Richard Simmons, you can choose a sensible exercise program that is right for you. Try as many different exercises as you have to until you find one that you enjoy. It's important to make sure that you make it fun. If it's a chore or you find it boring, forget it. If you don't like it, you won't do it. Don't throw in the towel too soon, though. Sometimes the first couple of days are the most difficult, and after that, it gets easier.

Of course, it always a good idea to consult your doctor before you begin to exercise. Get physical—get THIN.

KEEP MOVING FORWARD!

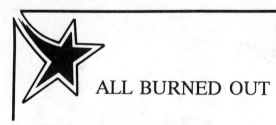

ALL BURNED OUT

All burned out? Just don't care? Feel frazzled and not able to love life?

Are you just dragging yourself out of bed or do you wake up every morning excited about the new day? Are you satisfied with life and ready to take on any new challenge that awaits you with delight? Why not? Truly, that is the way that life can be lived.

Do you put unreasonable pressures upon yourself by making your expectations too grand? Then, do you expect to realize your high hopes and eventually become frustrated, unhappy, and disappointed with the results when you don't? Does that lead you to lose sight of your dreams in your struggle to over-achieve? Are you then unwilling to accept a more realistic goal...and BURN OUT?

If your goal is to live life as a THIN person, then your goal must be realistic. Progress must replace the need for perfection. Learning must replace the desire for a fast weight loss. Remember your prime goal is to find long-term gratification.

Accept the best you can do...while you strive to be the best you can be. Achieve what you can and respect yourself for your achievements. Minimize your mistakes and maximize your joys.

No need to burn out on life. Give your goal enough time to happen. Trade in the impatience of the past for a growing process that will help you learn new techniques to cope with your future. Develop a real enthusiasm for life!

SET THE WORLD ON FIRE!

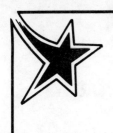

THE FORBIDDEN CITY

What made you FAT? Was it food? All foods or just certain foods? Do you acknowledge there are some foods that must be avoided forever? Are you convinced there is a FORBIDDEN CITY where you are not permitted to dwell?

The reason you are overweight is because you overeat...not because you eat the wrong foods. The reason you overeat has little to do with food. There are no BAD foods. However, letting go of your diet programming and learning to enjoy ALL foods can be frightening. Well, take heart...FOOD IS JUST FOOD.

Even though some foods may have been associated with negative behaviors in the past—and led to the destruction of your diets—they can become part of your life in the future. If you allow a mystique to prevail surrounding "forbidden foods"...you give them the power to control you.

Deprivation always leads to bingeing. However, if no foods are censored, they lose their power. Give yourself permission to eat ALL foods and your fear can be replaced with choice. Learn to control the foods you love. There is no need to deprive yourself ...enjoy yourself instead.

FOOD IS JUST FOOD. You can leave the FORBIDDEN CITY and live your life in freedom. No longer deprived...no longer bingeing...just eating in control.

SAY YES!

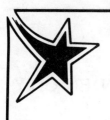

COLOR ME GREY

In the past, did you live your life in the world of black or the world of white? Were you either "gung ho" on a diet—or overeating with wild abandonment?

Did you faithfully divide foods into categories of "good" ...or "bad"?" Were you either "staying on a diet" or "cheating on a diet?" Did you eat cottage cheese, carrot sticks and unsweetened tea...or stuff yourself with anything with powdered sugar or chocolate sauce on it?

Did you live in two different worlds—deprivation or feasting? Were you saintly...or filled with guilt and self-hate? How about a middle ground?

Take heart, there are no "good" or "bad" foods. You no longer have to deprive yourself—or reward yourself—with food. The world is not black or white ...dieting or bingeing. Live in the lovely world of grey —the world of control! Make peace with food and your right to enjoy it.

Grey means the peace of loving yourself more than you love your food. Grey means never again facing the black despair of failure—or the stark whiteness of martyrdom in an effort to be THIN. Life is not black or white—it's a combination of both. Live peacefully in the THIN WORLD of grey.

MIX BLACK AND WHITE

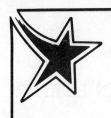

CELEBRATE
THE HOLIDAY!

Holiday time is to be celebrated. But, it is important to separate the nostalgia of the sights, smells, and memories of the past from the reality of the present.

Often holidays are tough to survive and enjoy because they are filled with a broad range of emotions. They can trigger memories of warm moments surrounded by family and friends...or memories of binge eating and self-loathing.

Make this year different. Enjoy the holidays to the fullest. If you are hungry for food...eat with gusto. If you are hungry for comfort...or pleasure...food is not the answer.

It is possible to enjoy the celebration without burying yourself in food. Be conscious of what you are eating and avoid deprivation. Before you get to the holiday table, have a positive strategy in mind. If your favorite foods are served, and you want to taste them—taste away! Sometimes a little bit of something satisfying is a whole lot better than a lot of nothing.

If you think that leftovers will create a control problem for you, give them to your guests as they are leaving—or throw them out! If you do lose the battle for control—when the holiday is over—return to your THIN LIFESTYLE and continue your journey to your ideal weight.

CELEBRATE YOUR THIN LIFE

A DEAR JOHN LETTER

Food, ever since I can remember, you have been my passion...my friend...my fun...my everything. You have been my bridge over troubled waters...my comfort when things go wrong...my best pal! So many times my desire for you has seemed uncontrollable and my thoughts of you have totally consumed me.

But, now I'm facing a harsh reality. Although your love has been so important to me in the past, the price tag is too high. True, you helped me bury all my sad feelings, but you also robbed me of my opportunity for joy.

Truth is you comfort me only while we are together because I hate myself once you are gone. Thanks for keeping me company when I've been lonely and for entertaining me when I've been bored—but, no thanks. You put my health at risk...steal my self-esteem...and tie my happiness to a number on a scale.

Food, because of you, my life has been a combination of despair, frustration and desperation. You've forced me to live with guilt, shame, and fear.

So, dear food...please be on notice that from this day forward, I love myself more than I love you. Therefore, I am ending our affair...it has to be over as I yearn to be free...free of you...free to be the best I can be...free at last!

FREE TO BE THIN!

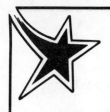

PROMISES...PROMISES...PROMISES

I promise that I am going to lose five pounds this week. I promise I am going to stay on my diet this time. I promise I am never going to have another binge. Promises...Promises...Promises...

I promise that when I get THIN, I am going to buy myself something new to wear. I promise when I get THIN, I am going to take better care of myself. I promise that when I get THIN, I am going to make new friends. I promise that when I get THIN, I am going to ask my boss for a raise. Promises...Promises ...Promises...

If being overweight is limiting your choices in life, make the commitment to change the patterns of your life. Why promise? Why wait? There is no time like the present and no reason to postpone life! Enjoy yourself NOW—by living life to its fullest—and not putting your dreams on hold because of your weight. Rather than promising to lose five pounds... promise to fight for control. Rather than promising to grind out another fad diet...practice choosing ALL foods in portion control.

What kind of life do you want for yourself? Start living it today by taking control of the rest of your life. You have everything you need to accomplish your dreams. Promise yourself, you are going to use it.

PROMISE YOURSELF A THIN LIFE!

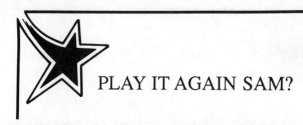

PLAY IT AGAIN SAM?

Your brain functions as the world's most sophisticated computer. Unfortunately, it has been programmed with "diet software." It is going to be necessary for you to change the notions of the past that have not served you very well—and replace them with THINK THIN programs.

For starters, FOOD IS JUST FOOD. It's appropriate use is to provide fuel for your body—not as a replacement for dealing with your emotional environment.

Perhaps in the past, in an effort to avoid dealing with difficult issues, you focused on food instead. Maybe you used food to "change the subject" when you did not wish to address the problem at hand. Well, no longer.

You've tried dieting and deprivation, but cursed yourself for your weakness and lack of willpower. Well, you are not to blame. Diets never work. It's true that dieting was all you knew, so you just kept playing the same old computer tapes over and over. Now, there is a new truth. So, don't play it again, Sam! Play a new tune...learning a new eating lifestyle, handling your problems without food, eating only when you are hungry and stopping when you've had enough.

Begin making the choices that will help you build success—one victory at a time. Soon your brain will be reprogrammed with a THIN LIFESTYLE. You will be playing a new tune....

SING A HAPPY SONG!

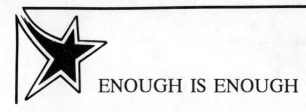

ENOUGH IS ENOUGH

What do you say to someone who keeps making the same mistakes? How do you treat someone who repeats the behaviors of the past over and over again? Do you assume that they do not wish to find success or that they do not know how to find success?

Have you ever been fooled by the ads on television, in the newspapers, and on the radio. Have you been the victim of products that promise magical weight losses?

The peddlers of these gimmicks only care about making a quick buck. They thrive on your desperation by bilking you for their expensive programs. They set you up for failure with their worthless weight loss schemes which only lead to the destructive cycle of losing and gaining weight. In addition, dangerous side effects can result in serious injury to your health.

Well, enough is enough! It's time to accept the fact that there is no brass ring on the diet merry-go-round. Diets lead only to misery...pain...and failure. But, who failed? You did not fail the DIET WORLD...it failed you!

You can learn from the past and not be doomed to relive it. Yesterday is gone...concentrate on today.

Promise yourself you will not be fooled again. You do not have to remain a helpless victim of greedy charlatans. Trying to lose weight FAST with the help of expensive diet "fads and gimmicks" can be replaced by slow and steady progress toward becoming a new YOU.

I'VE HAD ENOUGH!

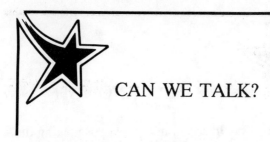

CAN WE TALK?

Can we talk? Boy, can we talk! Are you forever talking about food and losing weight? Do you know the details of every "fad" diet? Do you have a constant dialogue going about being overweight? Well, you are not alone.

Friends together for lunch are—while feasting, of course—talking about how much weight they want to lose. Dinner party conversation often centers around the latest fad diets and who's on it and how they're doing. Teenagers, obsessed by their weight, spend their lunch break talking about food and poking fun at anyone bigger than a size 5!

Television talk shows are never more popular than when they feature a guest who has written a new book about "quick" weight losses. Of course, they're popular. They give us something else to talk about.

Talk may be cheap, but it's not a very effective way to lose weight. The only way to truly get THIN and stay THIN is to make a commitment to live a THIN LIFESTYLE.

You have everything it takes to become a THIN person, so it's time to stop talking and START DOING! You can take control of your eating and take charge of your life. Then, as you get closer and closer to your ideal weight, your *silence* on the subject of dieting will be absolutely *golden*. And, when you reach your ideal weight...everyone will be talking about how great you look.

TALK ABOUT THIN!

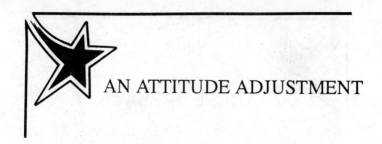

AN ATTITUDE ADJUSTMENT

I promise that I am going to lose ten pounds by my birthday. I swear I am never going to eat sweets again. I vow that I will never cheat again on my diet. Making unrealistic promises can be very self-defeating. So, why make promises?

Why not take one day at a time...making the best choices possible and learning how to eat like a THIN person? It's not the scale that is the measure of your success!

Throw out those diet books. Toss away the magazines that promise instant and unrealistic weight losses. Fad diets have never worked for YOU in the past...so, replace them with a new positive ATTI-TUDE!

Every time you make a promise and break it—every time you say, "I can't do it"—every time you feel that you blew it—you strengthen the negative attitude that has been keeping you FAT!

Instead, counter that negativity immediately with positive affirmations, "I can do it." "I will do it." "I am doing it."

Remember, a poor choice does not constitute a bad day...a bad week...a bad you! Use those choices as a learning experience. Let them help you to learn how to handle difficult situations in the future. It takes time to change lifelong habits, so use your new positive attitude to put you back on the track.

ADJUST YOUR ATTITUDE

207

REST IN PEACE

It's time to bury the past and let it rest in peace. Admittedly, it's painful to let go of your old emotional baggage, still, it must be done or it will hold you back from focusing on the future. Instead of feeling defeated over diet failures, and wallowing in times gone by, get to the heart of the obstacles standing in your path and remove them. Past disappointments—remnants of old hurts—or repressed angers—must all be resolved or dwelling on leftovers from the world of diets will retard your progress.

The first step toward a new start is to forgive and forget the past, yet respect its impact on the present. Don't put yourself down for having fears...don't blame yourself for wanting to turn back...just focus forward. The mistakes you made in the past are dead. Shifting into forward gear will allow you to become optimistic. The only thing that is important is what you will become in the future.

Change your self-defeating thinking and self-limiting attitudes from the past. Turn anxiety into challenge. Start with small steps forward and soon you will be leaping into the future. Courage is the ability to survive defeat, disappointment, and loss. Survive the past and create a new future.

GOOD-BYE YESTERDAY!

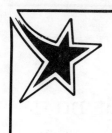

IF ONLY...

Do you have your desire to be THIN tied to the circumstances of your life? IF ONLY...my life was less hectic, I could lose weight. IF ONLY...I liked my job and my boss, I could lose weight. IF ONLY ...the baby wasn't sick and could go to nursery school, I could lose weight. IF ONLY...IF ONLY...IF ONLY...

Your environment, your emotional well-being, your troubles and pressures certainly do effect your ability to concentrate on losing weight. External pressures make the job tougher...but not impossible.

If you are waiting for the perfect time—when everything is running smoothly and life is without difficulties to lose weight—you may have a long wait!

Do it NOW. Plan a new way of life and avoid the pitfalls of the past, turn problems into challenges and despair into hope.

Tell yourself—IF ONLY...I believe that I can do it ...I can do it. Your life, your boss, your baby are not responsible for your weight—YOU ARE. Focus your mind on the new way you want your life to be and then concentrate on making it happen.

Have the courage to pursue your desire to be THIN—no matter what else is going on in your life. IF ONLY...you make a beginning...soon you'll be THIN.

WHY WEIGHT?

THE DEVIL MADE ME DO IT

"I just couldn't help myself." "I can't resist temptation." "I don't know why I did it." "Honestly, I tried!" Sound familiar?

After starting out with such wonderful intentions, what suddenly causes you to change your course of action?

I had a flat tire...*so, I had a whole pizza.* It was raining and I broke my umbrella...*so, I had a hot fudge sundae.* I locked my keys in the car...*so, I locked myself in a candy store.* My air-conditioner was broken...*so, I went into the pool with a pitcher of pina coladas.* I broke a fingernail...*so, I broke my diet.*

Since you begin with such a firm resolve—what happens? Is it the devil that makes you do it? Or, perhaps, you just surrender and give up your fight to win the war over food. Is it because you don't feel you are strong enough to resist?

Why surrender? You can give the devil a run for his money. Sure, in the past, you were a champion excuse maker. But, be honest...a trip to the refrigerator is no "Mr. Fixit." FOOD IS JUST FOOD! It is not a problem solver!

Sooo, tell FAT to go to the devil...and tell yourself that you can succeed.

GIVE 'EM HELL AND GET THIN!

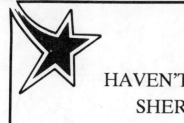

HAVEN'T A CLUE,
SHERLOCK!

You have departed on an exciting journey to your ideal weight. A travel diary can be a valuable asset. An accurate record of your positive and negative experiences can make you more conscious of your eating behaviors and thought patterns. Since you are looking for a long-term, permanent lifestyle change, your diary can help to make you aware of your negative habits. It can also act as your compass to point you in the direction of self-discovery.

If you detect that you nibble constantly while watching TV—or you binge when you are angry—or depression is the trigger for overeating—you have become aware of your previously unconscious eating patterns. Awareness of your actions is a giant step toward developing new ideas, attitudes, and concepts.

Keeping a diary can be like sharing your life with a friend that you love and trust. In addition, recording feelings with regard to problems and troubles often reduces the frustration and confusion surrounding them. Remember, though, this is a voyage to freedom—not a guilt trip! Your objective is to discover a whole new world. A world where you are comfortable about being you. How can you steer a course for your new world without a vision of the proper path to follow?

If your eating behavior is the crime—then you must become the detective to find the clues to solve the case.

ELEMENTARY...MY DEAR WATSON!

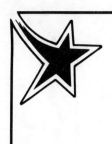

A SQUARE PEG

For years, overweight people have been treated like square pegs—trying to fit into the round hole of the THIN world!

You had to face the ridicule, disapproval, and the scorn of society. You had to deal with the condemnation of the DIET WORLD which claimed that you lacked willpower and the ability to control "forbidden" foods. You suffered discrimination, recrimination, and misery. You took the blame for failure because as each of your diets ended, you had learned nothing about being THIN. You were never taught to control "forbidden" foods or your programmed reaction to them. The issue of your emotional attachment to food was never addressed by your diet.

Trying to live in the THIN WORLD, without the essential information about being THIN, is like trying to put a square peg in a round hole. You have been kept in the dark long enough. Forget dieting, the fear of failure, ridicule, and scorn. Believing in your own self-worth and denying the responsibility for past diet failures is the way to become the well "rounded" person that you desire to be.

Have faith in yourself. Replace your doubts with positive thoughts. Replace fears and worries with self-trust. You are no longer a square peg in the FAT WORLD, but a new THIN you...who will fit in anywhere.

THIN AND WELL ROUNDED!

NICE GUYS FINISH FAT

There are many situations along your way to your ideal weight that are quite difficult. If you allow the behavior of others to influence or interfere with your determination, then you allow others to keep you FAT.

You may have to deal with some people who will purposely try to discourage your efforts by insisting that you are not being rewarded fast enough, "You worked that hard for only 1/2 pound?" Or, you may have to face a food pusher, who will insist, "But, it's a very special dinner and you can go right back on your diet tomorrow."

You may also have to deal with friends with whom you have always shared food and who may now feel rejected when food is rejected. Perhaps, you will encounter friends who envy what you are doing because they do not have the control to do it. Some friends may feel sorry for you because they fear you are depriving yourself. They want to give you permission to use food to make you happy.

Your response has to be strong. Put yourself on the top of your priority list. Refuse any offer that takes away your right to make your own choices and ONLY your own choices.

Speak up for your right to be THIN. Being too nice and wanting to please others at the expense of yourself will keep you from crossing the finish line in your race to your ideal weight.

NICE GUYS CAN FINISH THIN

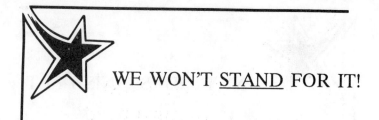

WE WON'T <u>STAND</u> FOR IT!

Think about how much extra you eat as your "standing operating procedure"...

While you are <u>standing</u> in the kitchen cooking, it's a taste of roast beef to see if it is done...a spoonful of rice to see if it's soft...a spoonful of soup to make sure that it's hot enough—and just to be sure—taste everything again!

<u>Standing</u> with the fridge open—just looking—often leads to picking on some chicken, nibbling on a slice of cheese, or discovering a piece of leftover cake.

While unpacking the groceries, if you <u>stand</u> around with a box of cereal or cookies in hand—before too long, you wind up with an empty box!

<u>Standing</u> in the kitchen just contemplating life could lead to sticking something in your mouth that you never intended to put there...go <u>stand</u> some place else.

There is no way to control portions if you are <u>standing</u> around and eating by the light of the refrigerator. Besides, it's unwise to ever eat anything out of its original container. Put all the food you intend to eat on a plate...even if you are only going to eat a carrot stick.

Change your habits and change your weight. Sooooo, remember, your best choices are made when you have planned for them..."sit down on the job".

<u>STAND</u> UP AND CHEER FOR THIN

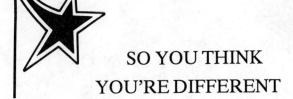

SO YOU THINK
YOU'RE DIFFERENT

Have you been on a diet since birth? Have you tried EVERYTHING...the liquids, powders, packaged foods? Do you feel faint at the sight of a beautiful cream pie? Have you ever met a pizza or a pasta that you didn't love?

Do you often feel that YOU and only YOU have been doomed to live a life where stepping on the scale is a major trauma?

Well, you are not alone! Sure, there are a few lucky souls who were born with a "magic metabolism," but truly, they are few and far between. THIN people simply have a different relationship with food —and so must you!

Sacrifices have to be made. Changes must occur. Portions must be controlled. Inappropriate eating behaviors have to be corrected. But, you can do it. It's tough, but it will be worth it when you reach your ideal weight.

Sure, you want a FAST and EASY weight loss. But, now the difference is that you know there is no FAST and EASY way to change the attitudes, behaviors, and expectations of the past. Losing weight ALONE is not enough unless it leads you to a permanent lifestyle change. You're building a new master plan for life—trading despair for hope. Your future looks bright.

So, stick with it. You are becoming a different person...a THIN one!

NOT DIFFERENT...JUST THIN!

DON'T RAIN ON
MY PARADE

Nobody can make you THIN so don't allow anyone to help make you FAT. Often it is the behavior of others that is allowed to be the determining factor in the choices that you make for yourself.

A well meaning hostess who insists "I made it just for you" and you are only too happy to eat what you don't need...even if you really don't want it.

Someone hurts your feelings and BANG...A BINGE! Someone insults you "You look like you gained weight" and BOOM...A BINGE!

A friend gives you permission to eat too much and OOPS...A BINGE! If it's a bad day...that's a good reason for a bad choice...WHY? Sure, it's tougher to make good choices when you are being sabotaged and don't have the support of others. Sure, there are some around you who feel it is their duty to make sure you don't succeed. If you do, then they would feel the need to succeed as well.

Of course, there is one person you can always count on...YOURSELF. However, if you have a sympathetic friend or relative, ask for help. Find someone who supports your efforts and encourages your endeavor to change. Make sure it is someone who will understand mistakes as well as successes. Then, take all the help they are willing to give.

LEAD THE THIN PARADE!

MY VERY BEST FRIEND

The way you feel about yourself is a major factor in your ability to change. Building self-confidence can be easy if you practice treating yourself with the same kind of respect that you show others. Speak kindly to yourself. You are worthwhile, deserving and entitled to happiness.

If something goes wrong—fix it. Don't berate yourself for a simple mistake or you can kill your motivation. Remember, you're not perfect, nor do you have to be. If something doesn't work out—don't give up! When things don't go your way—don't throw in the towel. Recommit yourself to the discipline needed to pursue your desire to reach your ideal weight—NO MATTER WHAT! You possess inner resources that you haven't even begun to tap into yet.

Be positive—it is the best way to handle negative situations. Forget yesterday and avoid the self-criticism of the past. Compliment yourself on how well you are doing today. Be quick to give yourself credit and reluctant to pile on blame. Appreciate yourself for making the decision to take control of your own destiny. You have the courage to survive disappointments. You have the determination to be THIN. Think positive thoughts about yourself. Everything in your life is determined by how you feel about yourself, so give loving yourself a chance. After all, you've never had a better friend. A good mood and a terrific attitude are your best strategies for success.

I REALLY LIKE ME!

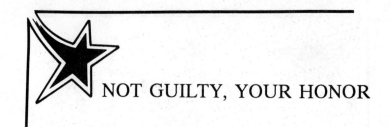

NOT GUILTY, YOUR HONOR

Guilt may have become such a part of your life that it is like your favorite shirt or an old shoe. You know that it is time to part with it...but, it is so comfortable that you just keep hanging on.

Some guilt is appropriate. It can alert you to situations that are wrong and allow you to make the proper corrections. However, inappropriate guilt diminishes self-esteem and produces a feeling of worthlessness. It robs you of your assertiveness and begins a pattern of self-destructive behavior.

For dieters, guilt is almost an occupational hazard. Well, that can be changed. Guilt with regard to old food habits is truly inappropriate guilt. Mistakes happen! If you "blow it"... so what?. There are worse crimes in life than eating the wrong thing.

To avoid guilt feelings, do not censor any foods. Instead of dividing food into categories of "good" and "bad"—make peace with food—and with yourself.

Let making a mistake be a learning experience and not a guilt trip. Blaming yourself for being human is counter productive. Instead of concentrating on guilt feelings, focus on taking positive steps to correct your negative behaviors. That will serve you much better than punishing yourself with guilt.

Stop feeling guilty! Be realistic. It will take time to alter your attitude toward food...but, you are working on it!

GUILTY OF BEING HUMAN!

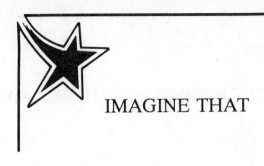

IMAGINE THAT

What is reality? Is it what you see or what you think you see? What is THIN? Do you find it in the mirror...on the scale...or in your attitude?

Imagine yourself on a fun trip to your ideal weight instead of suffering through another horrible diet. Imagine not worrying about what foods you can or cannot eat. Imagine not being concerned about how much weight you've lost in a week, but rather feeling pleased about how much you've learned in a week.

Imagine yourself as a THIN person—who cannot conceive a binge—who will never have to deal with another diet—who will live a THIN LIFESTYLE forever.

Imagine yourself having the control to handle all foods—making a selection in any restaurant—enjoying social events—and never suffering the frustration and desperation of being out-of-control.

Imagine yourself as the person that you have always wanted to be—in control of your feelings—of your food—and of yourself. Imagine honoring the commitment to be THIN and never having to face the fear of FAT again. Imagine never again suffering the heartache of guilt and shame—never again making excuses—never again the failure of dieting...NEVER AGAIN.

Imagine your success and make it a reality. What is reality? It is a wonderful new you...free to live life just as you have always imagined it could be.

FOR REAL...YOU CAN BE THIN!

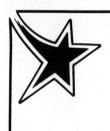

SUNNY SIDE UP

Expect the best and that is exactly what you are going to get! In the DIET WORLD you could never expect the best. Deprived of your right to self-determination and chastised for not being able to obtain perfection—you lived with guilt, shame and despair.

You can turn your worst pain into your hope for the future. You don't need any more information about dieting...it has never led you to success. Instead, if you expect to find your own way to success, there is absolutely no way you can fail. If you continue the pattern of deprivation and bingeing, THIN will always be beyond your reach.

It's time to accentuate the positive—I made the best choices possible...and I am proud of myself. I lost a half a pound this week...and I am proud of myself. It was tough to stay in-control...but I did it...and I am proud of myself.

Activate positive thoughts and combat the tendency toward negativity. If you slip up...forget it. Expect to make mistakes, correct them and continue. Forget yesterday and all the yesterdays when you did not succeed. Believe in yourself and in your ability to reach your ideal weight.

It is time to stop dwelling on what you can't eat and begin concentrating on what **YOU CAN DO**—and you can be THIN.

TURN IT AROUND AND BE THIN!

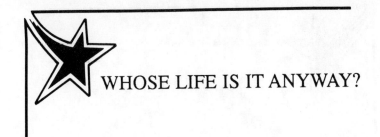

WHOSE LIFE IS IT ANYWAY?

Unfortunately along your way to becoming a new THIN person, there may be people in your life who will try to sabotage your efforts. Some unconsciously do the wrong thing, but others know exactly what they are doing. They don't want your success, probably because of jealousy or insecurity on their part.

Brace yourself! Get ready for comments like "You've lost enough already...you look so drawn." or "I really liked you better FAT."

Your mate or mother may not know how to deal with your new devotion to yourself. They may be frightened that the change in you will change how you feel about them. It's important to acknowledge their feelings and reassure them that your new food lifestyle won't affect your relationship with them.

Friends have a way of wanting us to share...share my fresh baked cake...share the dinner I made just for you. When you reject the food, they may feel that you are rejecting their friendship as well. Be positive and reassure them that their fears are groundless. Let them know the changes you are making in your life are positive and you are quite comfortable with the way you are eating—and your decision to live a THIN LIFESTYLE.

The only important issue is that YOU like YOU a whole lot better.

LIVE LIFE YOUR WAY!

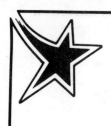

JUST SAY NO!

Have you ever been offered food when you didn't want it? Did anyone ever question your right to eat the foods you have chosen? Has anyone ever offered you a copy of their latest diet insinuating that you could really use it? What did you do?

When someone offers food that you don't want and don't need...just say "NO." It is not necessary to be polite and take food you don't want. Be honest! It's your right.

When someone asks if you are eating something you are not suppose to eat...just say "NO." You have the right to make your own choices.

When a person asks if you would like a copy of their latest diet...just say "NO." Well meaning or not, let people know that you don't appreciate their comments about your body. Don't allow anyone to hurt your feelings.

Get in touch with how you feel about the actions of others. Do you rebel and do the opposite? Do you cave in and surrender? Do you turn your anger at them toward yourself by bingeing? Do you assume they are right and you are wrong?

Saying "NO" when you mean "NO" is a valuable tool for dealing with every area of your life. Every time you say "NO" you feel better about yourself. Practice saying "NO" to others and "YES" to yourself.

SAY YES TO THIN!

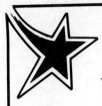

WHO'S THE BOSS?

For many years, perhaps, you have allowed food to be your BOSS. It decided WHAT you ate...WHEN you ate...WHY you ate...and HOW you ate. You have made a commitment to changing...to taking charge of your own choices...to becoming the BOSS. Now you can call your own shots!

Don't be afraid of a life without excess food. You can learn to eat when you are physically hungry and stop when you have had enough. You can establish control over food because FOOD IS JUST FOOD... and no more!

You can handle your life in a rational, non-emotional way and produce solutions that will work. You can form new habits to handle old situations... new attitudes toward old theories...new ways to cope with old problems.

Every time you give in to the compulsive urge to eat...food is the BOSS. Every time you fall back into the habit of dealing with your problems by overeating ...food is the BOSS. Every time you use a binge to escape reality...food is the BOSS. Success lies in the courage to take responsibility for your life. Focus your energy on defeating food and becoming the BOSS of your own life.

Remember you never fail until you stop trying and you never lose until you stop fighting! Sooooo, get BOSSY...get THIN.

YOU ARE THE BOSS!

IN THE STARS

Have you often thought that you were fated to be overweight? Did you think that FAT was your destiny—the luck of the draw? FAT is not a cruel joke of fate or a sentence to a lifetime of pain.

Maybe you have lived much of your life as a FAT person—dieting or overeating. Maybe you have NEVER found success before, but surely that does not mean that the Gods are against you.

There is no need to blame the stars, or curse the fates, or condemn yourself for your weight. It simply means you must accept NEW solutions to your OLD problems.

You are not a victim of fate. You have choices. Your life is not being controlled by some unknown destiny. You have the power to change your fate. You can jump off the vicious diet merry-go-round... and live the rest of your life in control.

The first step is to believe that luck has nothing to do with being THIN! It's not good luck that allows some people to be THIN and bad luck that leads to FAT. You have the opportunity to take command of your own life. That's right—control is yours for the taking.

You are the STAR of your life and a STAR is one who shines its own light—follows its own path—and shines the brightest in the darkness.

FOLLOW YOUR OWN STAR

AFTERWORD

I wrote DIET IS A 4 LETTER WORD in an effort to help end the suffering of being overweight. I've shared my victory hoping that, in some small way, it can inspire you to triumph.

I hope you will grab the opportunity to pursue your dream of living life as a THIN person. Don't stop here! Read on and learn all that you can about becoming the best you can be. The bookstores are stocked with great "self-help" books on a large variety of subjects. Professional therapy is another path you may choose to follow. Consider starting a support group in your neighborhood.

Your success is very important to me. I'd love to hear from you and hope you will share your progress with me. I wish you well.

Suzie Heyman
c/o The Thin Weigh
1893 N.E. 164th Street
N. Miami Beach, FL 33162